The Face: A Cultural Geography

Marty Roth

The Face: A Cultural Geography

Marty Roth

Academica Press
Washington~London

Library of Congress Cataloging-in-Publication Data

Names: Roth, Marty (author)
Title: The face : a cultural geography | Roth, Marty.
Description: Washington : Academica Press, 2022. | Includes references.
Identifiers: LCCN 2022940215 | ISBN 9781680537505 | 9781680537512 (e-book)

The Human face, that mirror of the Deity, that master-piece of the visible creation.

Johann Kaspar Lavater

For who knows *what a face is*, and is our notion thereof not mere prejudice, a limitation of the staggering number of forms that could constitute a face in their inexhaustible combinations?

Rainer Maria Rilke

Like a novel, the face is a web of living meanings, an inter-human event, in which the thing and its expression are inextricably joined.

Maurice Merleau-Ponty

The possibility of drawing near to the . . . face is the primary originality and the distinctive quality of the cinema.

Ingmar Bergman

The face possessed a magical significance around the time of massive popularity of magazines like Life or Vogue, when as Barthes says, "capturing the human face still plunged audiences into the deepest ecstasy, when one literally lost oneself in a human image as one would in a philter, when the face represented a kind of absolute state of the flesh, which could be neither reached nor renounced"

Teresa Brus

What is this thing, this structure of skin and bone and gristle and muscle, that we are condemned to carry around with us wherever we go? Where does it begin, where does it end? And why does everyone see it rather than seeing me?

J. M. Coetzee

Contents

Introduction

Man is read in his face; God in His creatures.
Ben Jonson, *Discoveries.*

In the Indian legend of "The Face of Glory," Shiva creates a ravenously hungry half-lion to do his bidding. When an intended victim is pardoned, the lion begs the god to provide him with food.

> Whereupon Shiva, with one of those inspirations such as occur only to the greatest, suggested that the monster should eat himself—to which work the prodigy immediately turned and the gorgeous banquet began. Commencing with his feet and hands, continuing through his legs and arms, the monster, ravenous and unable to stop, let his teeth go right on chopping through his belly, chest, and even his neck, until there was nothing left but a face. And the god, who had been watching with delight this epitomization of the self-consuming mystery that is life, smiled, when the feat had been accomplished . . . and said to it: "You shall be known henceforth as Kirttimukha, 'Face of Glory,' and shall abide forever at my door" (Campbell 218).

This book will not be about lions but about humans–human faces (1). In fact, much discourse insists that animals do not have faces, and it is the having of a face that makes one human. "How is it," Norbert Elias asks, "that, of all animals, man alone has developed a face so mobile, so infinitely variable, and, as we say, expressive that those of all other organisms appear by comparison masklike?" (302-3). And that face is also unified: it is not simply an assemblage of features but "the singularity of an impression" (Benson 32). It is also the site on which identity markers (of gender, ethnicity and age) display themselves, the body part that most pointedly allows the subject to be named and located in a history. The face, Kōbō Abe declares, is my copyright. It is unique; no two faces are identical. And the loss of face suffered by veterans and accident victims is usually regarded as a loss of their humanity.

The face is usually taken to be the proper representation of the person behind it; "Look at me" means "look at my face." According to Plato, the head is the divine part of us which controls the rest, the "acropolis" of the body; the body is there just to move the head around and protect it (*Timaeus*). It is the site of four of our five senses, the inlet for eating and drinking, the inlet and outlet for breathing, as well as the reservoir of judgments as to our beauty or ugliness. "Whoever falls in love, briefly or lastingly, in earnest or light heartedly, falls in love, almost always with a face" (Belting 2). The face is also our social dimension, "the only location of community" (Agamben 2000:91).

That face, that human center, is also a measurable surface, one that can be mapped for purposes of identification, containment and punishment. As Alan Sekula says, "Every proper portrait has its lurking, objectifying inverse in the files of the police;" even worse, as Roland Barthes and Friedrich Kittler note, "the Photomat always turns you into a criminal type, wanted by the police;" "On identification photos, one sees only the faces of criminals not because the media lie, but because they fragment the narcissism of one's own conception of the body" (Sekula 14, Barthes 12 and Kittler 93). In *Gravity's Rainbow* Thomas Pynchon asks the reader: "Is that who you are, that vaguely criminal face on your ID card, its soul snatched by the government camera as the guillotine shutter fell?" (134).

As such, the face is also a biopolitical prison, a key feature in the program of late capitalism--photographed, stored and used to certify identity. Technology claims to be able to efficiently identify and process faces to service "an explosively emerging 'global face culture,' exemplified by biometrics and facial detection technologies, driven by ever obsessive and paranoid impulses to know, capture, calculate, categorize, and standardize human faces":

> . . . security technology for border crossings and visas, invasive surveillance cameras in urban settings, biometric marketing and enormous biometric data gathering sweeps; and the facial identification and verification platforms found in social media and consumer markets, "from Facebook's auto-face-tagging to the iPhone's RecognizeMe application that uses face scanning to unlock phones" (Blas) (2).

Contemporary culture is marked by the incessant circulation of the face as an element of public exchange, featuring a cult of celebrity faces (actors, dancers, politicians, generals) that intrude into our private lives: "The movie stars and matinee idols are put into the public domain by photography. They become dreams that money can buy. They can be bought and thumbed more easily than public prostitutes" (McLuhan). Lady Wotton informs Dorian Gray that she recognizes him because of the ubiquity of his face: "I know you quite well by your photographs. I think my husband has got twenty-seven of them," she says. Dorian retorts, "Not twenty-seven, Lady Henry?" "Well, twenty-six then." In the contemporary urban landscape the face we see endlessly replicated is our own: in store windows, mirrors and video images. In Stephen Spielberg's "Minority Report," John Anderton (Tom Cruise) walks through a mall where he is bombarded with ads that hail him by name as they offer their products. While the video displays do not literally mirror him they use facial recognition technology to offer him a personalized consumer profile (3). And the face also circulates in a "small invasive cartoon army of faces," the more than three thousand emojis at our disposal; the OED's "Word of the Year" for 2016 was not a word, but a pictograph: the "Face with Tears of Joy" emoji (Gitelman). We look to the world for faces and few facelike features are needed for something to appear to us as a face: "There is a kind of blind desperation to our desire to see faces and to read them as expressive of mental states" (James Elkins in Carrier 93) (4). The face also has power: from Dante's Beatrice to Michel Hazanavicius's Bérénice.

Bernadette Wegenstein, however, gestures toward a post-facial regime:

> The face, which has always overcoded other body parts, has now ceased to be the most representative signifier of human appearance . . . every organ has an (inter)face; potentially, every organ may stand in for the whole body . . . . That is why, in current advertisements for beauty products, we see legs, arms, or whole bodies in action, and almost no classic portraits of faces anymore (2002:222 and 234).

Stephen Jaeger tells us that "A philosophy of the face, a phenomenology or a hermeneutics of facial expression, does not exist" (68). That may be so but there are certainly interesting and significant explorations of the topic--by Gilles Deleuze, Emmanuel Levinas, Jean-Luc Nancy, Robert Sobieszek and Jenny Edkins to name only a few. And Elias forecasts the failure of this book: "The variability of the human face is so great, the possible configuration of features so diverse, and the continuous changes in the landscape even of a single living face so manifold that our verbal equipment often falls short of our requirements if one tries, in words, to do justice to what one perceives" (303).

My chapters are pretty regular stations in the discourse: after the face itself, the mask and the veil; mirror recognition and misrecognition; the broken face of modern warfare and modern art; ugliness and beauty; and the mouth open in laughter and a scream. Strings of binary oppositions are woven through the chapters: the physiognomy of Lavater versus the pathognomy of Georg Christoph Lichtenberg (fixed features as opposed to the expressive play of the face), the buccal versus the oral mouth of Jean-Luc Nancy and the facial ethics of Levinas versus the faciality of Deleuze (a transcendental call to ethics as opposed to a systemic construction of white supremacy) among others.

The first chapter treats expression, both as revealing or concealing "the inner self," the generic faces of Francis Galton, the erasure of the face that follows upon urban living, ethnic physiognomy–the face of the Jew, the criminal, the queer--and the comparative physiognomy of humans and animals.

Francis Bacon's portraits are interrogations of the limits of the self. "Up to what degree of distortion," Milan Kundera writes, "does an individual still remain himself? To what degree of distortion does a beloved being still remain a beloved being? For how long does a cherished face growing remote through illness, through madness, through hatred, through death still remain recognizable?" (12) (5).

The face and the mask should be in opposition to one another, but they are regularly confounded and exchanged. Why do we need or want a second face? The mask is prominent in modern art (James Ensor, Pablo Picasso). There is also a special category of mask, the life and death mask, where the cover resembles the face. The constructed use of the face is also figured as a mask by Friedrich Nietzsche, Rainer Maria Rilke, Carl Jung or Erving Goffman. Cosmetics are also said to constitute a mask. Veils and masks have both come into political prominence recently, the first via hijab bans in Western states and the second through the Zapatista and Occupy movements in Mexico and the United States and, most recently, through the public health arena. The chapter ends with the veil as the dividing mark in the clash of civilizations.

The chapter on misrecognition moves from the face to the face-to-face and touches on the concept of likeness. Since we cannot see our faces, we must receive them from a likeness, most often the mirror reflection--and this transmission may even extend to our sense of self. On the other hand, as Gerald Bruns writes, "My face is not the locus of my self-identity: it is my shadow, a surplus me, an alter ego that exposes me to the world—to myself and to others in it;" mirrors alter and distort in various ways (585). Likeness is also disseminated through portraiture, photography and the cinematic closeup. Among the works discussed in this chapter are *The Picture of Dorian Gray*, "William Wilson," *Confessions of a Justified Sinner*, "The Secret Sharer," *The Comedy of Errors*, *Face/Off* and *Eyes Without a Face*.

The disfiguration and disappearance of the face in art and literature (already in process before the war) was stimulated by the high incidence of facial wounding in World War One. The broken faces of this war were transferred to text in Germany (in the form of New Objectivist art), displaced in France and Italy (emerging most prominently in Surrealism) and suppressed in England (with the possible exception of Francis Bacon) until the novels of Pat Barker and Louisa Young.

Another path led to the replacement of the human body by a doll, the department store mannequin, the dressmaker's dummy or the robot--figures with bland and empty faces. An earlier facial regime of disfigurement (in Victor Hugo, Robert Louis Stevenson, H. G. Wells or Stephen Crane, for example) consisted of faces that could not be described, could not be looked at or were asserted to have gone missing. The lost face was the one put forward by Deleuze and Giorgio Agamben: not a biological given, but a semiotic formation, a carapace affixed to (or projected onto) the head.

In the chapter on beauty and ugliness, the archetype of beauty and the beast poses the central question of this dialectic, can they breathe or dance together, can they coexist? Beginning as a nothing, then a foil to the beautiful, ugliness slowly came to play a part in aesthetics and eventually dominated that scene. But what, after all, is ugliness? Is it excess or contagion? It is paired off with cousin concepts like the monstrous and the grotesque and regularly contrasted with the sublime. Recently, beauty and ugliness have shifted from good and bad to old and new: new art is always ugly. Ugliness is regularly inflected as feminine–in the mythology of Medusa and the medieval "Loathly Lady" tales.

Of the many parts of the face–five holes, the eyes, nostrils and mouth; two extensions, ears and nose--I have chosen to treat only the mouth in any detail. I particularly wanted to avoid a chapter on the nose, because the subject has been thunderingly closed by Freud's penis equation and European antisemitism. The chapter on the mouth treats the history of smiling (particularly in its relationship to consumer capitalism); the gaping mouth; the buccal as opposed to the oral mouth; and the aestheticization of taste. The primary smiling and screaming objects in it are Hugo's "man who laughs," the Joker, the screamers of Edvard Munch and Francis Bacon and cinematic "scream queens."

"And are they parts," Socrates asks in *The Protagoras*, "in the same sense in which mouth, nose, and eyes, and ears, are the parts of a face; or are they like the parts of gold, which differ from the whole and from one another only in being larger or smaller?" But the former parts have a way of sliding into the latter, for, like the eyes, the smile also came to be viewed in the eighteenth century as a symbol of an individual's innermost and most authentic self and held to reveal the character of the person within (Colin Jones).

There are interesting stories to tell about those parts: of the anti-physiognomy of Michel Foucault where tears are not idle, but legible as a confession in the creation of the body's domesticity; of the kiss as a declaration of sexual desire as a modernist invention brought into prominence by the domestic ideology of Western cinema (under the Hollywood Code it was, for many years, the only sexual image allowed on screen); of spit as "a parodic alternative to spirit" in the counter-history of sovereignty; and of the Japanese tongue-lickers, a tall, bony creature with frilly hair and an extraordinarily long tongue, who leaves stains on the ceilings of houses, temples and shrines (Richman 59 and Foster).

The face circulates through most of the things of this world: anything that has presence, that presents itself, that has a front, a surface, an appearance, an aspect, reputation, honor, writing (as in type face)–anything that confronts, opposes or defies--has a face. And the face is a front: from the back it is just a head, a radically different entity according to Deleuze. My search engine turned up nearly as many instances of "facing something," "faced with" and "on the face of" as of face.

* * * * * * * * * * * * *

This is my fifth example of what I call discursive ethnography (or, in this case, cultural geography). As with the others (on memory, privacy, water and change), I acknowledge the abundance of quotation and the

Eurocentricity, almost without apology.

As Michel de Montaigne wrote in his essay on physiognomy:

> Without pains and without learning, having a thousand volumes about me in the place where I write, I can presently borrow, if I please, from a dozen such scrap-gatherers, people about whom I do not much trouble myself, wherewith to trick up this treatise of Physiognomy; there needs no more but a preliminary epistle of a German to stuff me with quotations.

What an historian like Fernand Braudel abjures–"all these soundwaves bouncing back and forth, jostling and interfering with one another"-- this cultural geographer glories in (Maglaque 29). So much has been written on these topics that I have chosen to let earlier works speak for themselves as much as possible.

I ran out of available colleagues decades ago. Thankfully my best reader is still around.

Facials 1

"I shouldn't know you again if we did meet," Humpty Dumpty replied in a discontented tone . . . "you're so exactly like other people."
"The face is what one goes by, generally,"
Alice remarked in a thoughtful tone.
"That's just what I complain of," said Humpty Dumpty. "Your face is the same as everybody has—the two eyes, so—" (marking their places in the air with this thumb) "nose in the middle, mouth under. It's always the same. Now if you had the two eyes on the same side of the nose, for instance—or the mouth at the top—that would be some help."
"It wouldn't look nice," Alice objected. But Humpty Dumpty only shut his eyes and said "Wait till you've tried."
Lewis Carroll, *Through the Looking-glass.*

Lady Macbeth likened her husband's face to "a book where men/ May read strange matters." "I see sold up in your face, George, as plain as print," Mrs. Bagnet says to Mr. George in *Bleak House*, and, in *Return of the Native*, Thomas Hardy writes of Clym Yeobright that "The observer's eye was arrested, not by his face as a picture, but by his face as a page; not by what it was, but by what it recorded."

According to Georg Christoph Lichtenberg, "We can see nothing whatsoever of the soul unless it is visible in the expression of the countenance . . . . As the magnet arranges iron filings, so the soul arranges around itself the facial features" (Fara 30). Physiognomists from Aristotle to Montaigne, Lavater and Cesare Lombroso tried to read the mind and heart as it was exhibited in the face: "For there are mystically in our faces certain Characters that carry in them the motto of our Souls," Sir Thomas Browne wrote, "wherein he that cannot read *A.B.C.* may read our natures." "Every human face" Arthur Schopenhauer said "is a hieroglyph which can be deciphered . . . man's face says more, and more interesting things than his mouth . . . It is a monogram of all man's thoughts" (232). The *Encyclopaedia Britannica* for 1853-60 noted that "In many places, where the study of human character from the face became an epidemic, the people went masked through the streets" (Graham 298).

Reading the face was quite a straightforward matter as Lavater presented it. He summarized the dialectic of beauty and ugliness as "The morally best, the most beautiful. The morally worst, the most deformed" (99). *Look ere You Leap*, a text that guided men in their selection of a wife, proposed that "a lovely fair Face does generally prove the Index of a fairer Mind" (Woods 144). The theory and practice of face-reading begins in antiquity, and there is a steady trail of observations through the ages. The passage by Lavater quoted earlier is a repetition of Baldassare Castiglione: "The ugly are therefore for the most part wicked too, and the beautiful are good: and we may say that beauty is the pleasant, gay, acceptable and desirable face of good, and that ugliness is the dark, disagreeable, unpleasant and sad face of evil." Physiognomists also read the future achievements of the individual in the face.

At the hands of James Hogg and Edgar Allan Poe, physiognomy became a technique close to mind-reading. Hogg says of his devil figure Gil-Martin:

> I observed several times, when we were speaking of certain divines and their tenets, that his face assumed something of the appearance of theirs; and it struck me, that by setting his features into the mould of other people's, he entered at once into their conceptions and feelings.

Poe's version is from "The Purloined Letter":

> When I wish to find out how wise, or how stupid, or how good, or how wicked is any one, or what are his thoughts at the moment, I fashion the expression of my face, as accurately as possible, in accordance with the expression of his, and then wait to see what thoughts or sentiments arise in my mind or heart, as if to match or correspond with the expression. (1)

The need for such a discipline became particularly acute in the eighteenth century as a result of urban crowding and a revolution in clothing that blurred clear markers of class and breeding. Physiognomy was a response to this bewildering flux of anonymous faces. Unfortunately, as Roy Porter convincingly argues, the practice fell under suspicion just when it was most needed. Lavater's work represents a resurrection of physiognomy as eighteenth-century cynicism gave way to the cultivation of sensibility in the

Pre-Romantic era. The narrator of Poe's "The Man in the Crowd" sits in a London coffeehouse, observing the dense crowds of people passing by the large bow window. He easily identifies the character and occupations of almost all the passersby when an old man "arrested and absorbed my whole attention, on account of the absolute idiosyncrasy of . . . [his face's] expression. Any thing even remotely resembling that expression I had never seen before . . . . Then came a craving desire to keep the man in view--to know more of him." (2) The actuary in Charles Dickens's "Hunted Down" installs a "thick plate glass" in his office "in order that I might derive my first impression of strangers, who came to us on business, from their faces alone, without being influenced by anything they said."

Like Lavater, Emanuel Levinas assumed a transparency between outside and inside. For both, the face is not only natural but transcendental. Looking at it, both of them see God. A passage early in *Totality and Infinity* identifies the face of the other ("The way in which the other presents himself, exceeding the idea of the other in me") as an epiphanic experience, "like stumbling upon an unexpected crevasse in the surface of the world" (Levinas 1991:50 and Moore 25). This encounter calls the self into being; it is the foundational moment of philosophy as well as the crux of social engagement. It leads to an ethical absolute: "Once I see the face of the other, I am automatically and infinitely obliged to it . . . . To see a face is already to hear 'You shall not kill'"–although, as Judith Butler notes, it is much more common to be presented with faces (like those of Sadam Hussein or Osama Bin Laden) and hear "kill!" (Levinas 1990:8-9 and Butler 141) (3).

What is it that the face is expressing? What lies beneath? Nathaniel Hawthorne's "inmost Me" or Shakespeare's "that within which passes show"–what we think of "commonsensically as being 'inside' the face, or behind or beneath it (the internal, intention, the signified, the impression, content, the cause of superficial signification effects, the substrate, and so forth)" or "whatever it may be called–personality, individuality, self, soul, character, 'invariant of consciousness' or software–what persists of being human [that] continues to be found embedded within, lurking behind, projected upon, or subsiding beneath the human face" (Cante 117 and Sobieszek 15)?

"Is the face singular or plural? Although no two faces may be alike, the face is also alleged to have generic properties: it belongs to a family, to a nation and more": "His face, person, and voice, were so exactly those of his father in his best days, that Glossin . . . almost thought the grave had given up its dead! (*Mannering*)." In his poem "Heredity," Hardy called it the "family face"

> I am the family face;
> Flesh perishes, I live on,
> Projecting trait and trace
> Through time to times anon.

Living in cities, according to sociologists, rubs out the face, as in a Bacon painting; faces in the city begin to resemble one another. Ernst Junger found that in urban dwellers "the tremendously homogeneous and typical aspects" of facial expressions were gaining the upper hand (Belting 82). Walter Benjamin believed that as capitalism came of age, people lost the integrity of their identity and the human face lost the aura to which early photography had been the last witness; as Norma Desmond declared in *Sunset Boulevard*, "We had *faces* then!" If one wanted to see the authentic face of a nation, one would leave the city and search for it in the countryside. In *The Face of the German Volk*, Ema Lendvai-Dircksen argued that "the peasant represented traditional values, and she juxtaposed this allegedly more authentic face against those of the alienated, modern urban world" (Brückle).

There was also an ethnic physiognomy which, in the case of the Jew, Proust called "racial eczema." *Out* Magazine wrote of a "gay face," a "set of recognizable gay facial characteristics and/or a propensity among gay men . . . to recognize (other) men who are gay 'by face alone'" (Cante 112). The turn-of-the-twentieth-century polymath Francis Galton devoted himself to the production of such composite faces (the criminal, the Jew etc.) through photography: "This photographic impression of an abstract, statistically defined, and empirically nonexistent criminal face was both the most bizarre and the most sophisticated of many concurrent attempts to marshall photographic evidence in the search for the essence of crime" (Sekula 19). Comparative physiognomy was a study of similarities between humans and animals; it had its roots in (pseudo)Aristotle's famous syllogism: lions are courageous, this man has the lion's features, therefore this man is courageous. Joseph Addison laid out the belief in Spectator No. 86: "As a Man hath in the Mould of his Face a remote Likeness to that of an Ox, a Sheep, a Lion, an Hog, or any other Creature; he hath the same Resemblance in the Frame of his Mind, and is subject to those Passions which are predominant in the Creature that appears in his Countenance." And Honoré de Balzac sets this equation up for the title character of his tale, "Z. Marcas":

> A common superstition has it that every human countenance resembles some animal. The animal for Marcas was the lion. His hair was like a mane, his nose was short and flat; broad and dented at the tip like a lion's; his brow, like a lion's, was strongly marked with a deep median furrow, dividing two powerful bosses. His high, hairy cheek-bones, all the more prominent because his cheeks were so thin, his enormous mouth and hollow jaws, were accentuated by lines of tawny shadows.

The theory is acted out in H. G. Wells's *The Island of Dr. Moreau* where "the human mark distorted but did not hide the leopard, the ox, or the sow, or other animal or animals, from which the creature had been moulded." But whereas the traditional physiognomical tradition acknowledges a seemliness in this transition, Wells makes the overlay repulsive: "Imagine yourself surrounded by all the most horrible cripples and maniacs it is possible to conceive, and you may understand a little of my feelings with these grotesque caricatures of humanity about me."

As opposed to Levinas, Deleuze and Félix Guattari (D/G) reject the tendency to see the face as an index of that which lies within or above, and they also "wish to divest the face of any auratic or seductive power of the kind that contemporary media–cinema, advertising, television–confer upon it"–although it is not clear exactly what face D/G and Levinas are theorizing (Conley 102). D/G work against common sense as usual; their theory repeatedly questions the notion of a coherent subject. Their *face* is imported from elsewhere, imposed on the head by an abstract process they call "faciality," a process that coincides with the formation of subjectivity. Facialization begins with the production of binary units-- white or black, straight or gay, mad or sane–that allow the face to be identified and seen as individual. It does not belong to the body (D/G make a clear distinction between the face and the head). Bacon, for example, is a painter of heads not faces, "and there is a great difference between the two. For the face is a structured, spatial organization that conceals the head, whereas the head is dependent upon the body, even if it is the point of the body, its culmination" (Deleuze 2002:15). The face was acquired at some point in the past and it is something that schizophrenics can lose.

Faciality presents itself as a system of surfaces and holes: a white wall with black holes in it. The face "brings together a despotic wall of interconnected signifiers (the horizon of paranoics who believe they can detect a master signifier behind the onslaught of signs) and passional black holes of subjective absorption" (Tamboukou 81). The despotic facial machine gives priority to the white wall and signification; while the authoritarian facial machine gives priority to the black holes and subjectification. The two, of course, mix and function together. The white wall acts like a movie screen, printing out a constant scroll of signification; the black holes of eyes and mouth seduce us into a mirage of subjectivity, into a passionate depth inhabited by the inmost Me (6).

The Deleuzian face is denied to "primitives, who wear mask-like surfaces. This face is not universal; It is white man himself, with his broad white cheeks and the black hole of his eyes" (D/G 1987: 176). This face was an invention of Western Christian Europe and designed to subordinate non-white, non-European faces; it was essentially the face of Christ, "the mask of the White Man par excellence, Jesus Christ superstar" (Herzog 70). Eastern and Western Christianity split over Jesus's face. In Constantinople, its representation was forbidden, while for Rome the face would be endlessly repeated and adored: "For the Christian world, from that moment on, the theology of the face is the key to power" (Ford 207).

"Speak that I may see thee," Socrates says in *The Charmides*.

If there is no face until there is signification for Deleuze, there is no face until there is language for Giorgio Agamben. Animals do not have a face: only humans want to seize hold of their own "being-manifest;" language is the appropriation which transforms nature into face. But the face not only speaks, it writes: as Dante struggles up Mount Purgatory he meets a "crowd of souls, silent and devout," the Gluttonous, with desiccated faces. "'The sockets of their eyes seemed like rings without gems,' and so the word *omo* (man) could be read easily on their faces. This refers to a medieval commonplace whereby the eyes were thought to form two O's, while an M was formed by the line of the eyebrows and nose" (Moore 25). Actually it is "*omo dei*"--the ears, nostrils and mouth forming the D, E and I (Synnott 1989:622). Nicholas of Cusa maintained that every human face is an image of the face of God: "So I see, oh Lord, that your face precedes every visible face, that it is the truth and the model of all faces." This divine stamp was obscured by the influence of sin, which caused "the defacing of that image and the destruction of that divine impress which had been formed when we were first created" (Moore 26 and 29).

Plutarch says that Cassander, one of the captains of Alexander, trembled all through his body when he saw a portrait of his King (Woodall 8). From God down through Christ, certain faces have extraordinary, iconic power, like the Mandylion, a piece of cloth on which the face of Jesus had been imprinted, or the Veil of Veronica, another piece of cloth, which, according to tradition, bears his likeness: Saint Veronica encountered Jesus on the Via Dolorosa on the way to Calvary and when she paused to wipe the blood and sweat from his face with her veil, his image was imprinted on the cloth. The face of Dante's Beatrice has redemptive power. The Western cinema of D. W. Griffith was constructed to display the power of the female face, as manifested in the close-up.

But what on our face is sending the messages signaling character? Is it the fixed features, as Lavater insisted, or the wide and shifting range of expressiveness that plays over our faces, as Lichtenberg, Lavater's harshest critic, declared (This binary is often expressed as countenance opposed to face; while Balázs linked fixed physiognomy to "inherited racial properties" and facial expressions to the tendencies of an individual soul)? (Carter 66). For those in the camp of Lavater, "Expression was distinguished from physiognomy: the former was about the temporary effects of the emotions on the face; the latter concerned those permanent facial features that revealed character" (West 34). The Italian polymath Giovanni Battista della Porta anticipated Lavater when he asserted that as the face represented "one's entire countenance, just as it does one's movements, and passions," it was necessary to judge it only "after the soul's emotions and passions have cooled." (Woods 140). Buffon and Darwin, however, wrote "against a tradition of physiognomic analysis which attributes character traits to the structure of the face rather than to its habitual movements" (Frow 236).

> In respect of character a face may make certain admissions by its outline; but it fully confesses only in its changes. So much is this the case that what is called the play of the features often helps more in understanding a man or woman than the earnest labors of all the other members together . . . . Eustacia's features went through a rhythmical succession of them. She glowed; remembering the mendacity of the imagination, she flagged; then she freshened; then she fired; then she cooled again. It was a cycle of aspects, produced by a cycle of visions (Hardy, *Return*).

Lichtenberg opposed "pathognomy" (reading character from

expressive behavior) to the former's physiognomy, although he acknowledged that repeated formations could leave a permanent record on the face. Facial expression, Abe wrote, "'comes like the annual growth rings in a tree trunk,' leaving their trace in habitual muscular response and in wrinkles, a historical record of the repeatable past" (Brilliant 111).

Charles Le Brun, a seventeenth-century art theorist, called the face an "instrument board," a fixed spectrum of expressions serving a fixed repertoire of affective states, and he identified the facial configuration for each passion (Gombrich 3). The face is a platform for the play of expressions that appear suddenly and vanish or morph into others. The face is so active that often its mobility alone is apparent; Lacan, for example, refers to it as a totally fluid entity, the most elusive of objects–a *perpetuum mobile*; Gerhard Richter also praises "the incredible and monstrous mobility of the face" (Magli 87 and Simmel in Richter 110). Faces change constantly over time ("I was certainly in earnest, and you seemed equally so," replied Hilda, glancing back at Donatello, as if to reassure herself of the resemblance. "But faces change so much, from hour to hour, that the same set of features has often no keeping with itself; to an eye, at least, which looks at expression more than outline"), altered, according to Proust, by their own history: "And just as, before kissing Odette for the first time, he had sought to imprint upon his memory the face that for so long had been familiar, before it was altered by the additional memory of their kiss."

With its eighty mimetic muscles, the face is capable of over 7,000 expressions. Addison played out this conceit in another *Spectator* paper: "Every Passion gives a particular Cast to the Countenance, and is apt to discover itself in some Feature or other. I have seen an Eye curse for half an Hour together, and an Eye-brow call a Man Scoundrel. Nothing is more common than for Lovers to complain, resent, languish, despair, and die in dumb Show."

The systematic mapping of expressions was undertaken in the nineteenth century by Charles Bell, Duchenne De Boulogne and Charles Darwin. Bell claimed that the muscles of the face were divinely designed to express uniquely human feelings; William A.F. Browne ridiculed Bell's theological explanations, pointing instead to the striking similarities of human and animal biology. Duchenne combined electricity and photography in his investigation of the mechanism of facial expression, producing a "semantics of facial muscular movement," a "a mosaic of muscles" which replaced the "muscular mask" that was the dominant scientific paradigm (Geroulanos). Forty-five years later (1872), Darwin revisited this issue, using Duchenne's map of the facial mechanisms. He reduced the number of commonly observed emotions from Duchenne's more than sixty to just six core expressions: anger, fear, surprise, disgust, happiness and sadness.

II

Momus, the Greek god of satire, thought that humans should have windows into their hearts so that their secret feelings could be discerned. Tristram Shandy wishes this were so:

> . . . had the said glass been there set up, nothing more would have been wanting, in order to have taken a man's character, but to have taken a chair and gone softly, as you would to a dioptrical bee-hive, and look'd in,—view'd the soul stark naked;—observed all her motions,—her machinations;—traced all her maggots from their first engendering to their crawling forth;—watched her loose in her frisks, her gambols, her capricios; and after some notice of her more solemn deportment, consequent upon such frisks, &c.——then taken your pen and ink and set down nothing but what you had seen, and could have sworn to.

In severing the body from the self, Descartes had also separated an inner reality accessible by reason from the appearances of the outside, and this division undermined faith in physiognomy throughout the eighteenth century. The villains of this period, Blifil, Fainall, Joseph Surface, Peachum or Jonathan Wild are all artful men adept at hiding their evil natures (7).

For Agamben, "The face is at once the irreparable being-exposed of humans and the very opening in which they hide and stay hidden;" the face is a "*mask that fails*, a surface haunted by intimations of concealment" (Agamben 90 and Coates 2). A face that "no longer discloses interiority," Jonathan Crary suggests, is already apparent as early as the 1860's in the works of Manet (92). "None will ever be a true Parisian," Gaston Leroux wrote, "who has not learned to wear a mask of gaiety over his sorrows and one of sadness, boredom or indifference over his inward joy."

Michael Taussig emphasizes the doubleness of the face as both mirror and mask (227). Our faces may reveal our thoughts and feelings or they may conceal them, hiding them behind some willfully simulated expressions; and expressions are regarded as extremely mobile–hence the idioms *take (or wipe) that expression off your face*. In the example of facial semiotics from Dickens that Richard Rushton uses to open his article "What Can a Face Do?" both true and false compete; the face is double-coded: "He saw a certain ambitious triumph in her face which no assumed coldness could conceal" (219). Levinas, as would be expected, opposes any interpretation of the face that would take it for a "mask dissimulating a real" and many writers believe that "micro leakages," as Paul Ekman terms them, seep through to reveal the emotional truth (Perpich 44) (9).

David Goldstein observes that "for Shakespeare the face is, foremost, a site of epistemological, ontological, and ethical crisis" (75). Hamlet tells us that "One may smile, and smile, and be a villain"–smile while something behind the smile seethes with hatred or resentment. In *3 King Henry VI*, Richard of Gloucester states:

> Why, I can smile, and murder whiles I smile,
> And cry "Content!" to that which grieves my heart,
> And wet my cheeks with artificial tears,
> And frame my face to all occasions. (3.2.182–185).

As a popular song of the forties put it: "I'm laughing on the outside, crying on the inside;" or as Victor Hugo wrote of the protagonist of *The Man Who Laughed*: "His face laughed. His thoughts did not. The exterior did not depend on the interior." William Hogarth wrote in *The Analysis of Beauty* that "The bad man, if he be a hypocrite, may so manage his muscles, by teaching them to contradict his heart, that little of his mind can be gathered from his countenance." Jean-Jacques Courtine dates this dynamic to the early modern period, "when self expression (the will to show the emotions) collided with self-control (the desire or compulsion to regulate the emotions)" (Belting 4).

The eighteenth-century code of "politeness" required expression to be managed for purposes of sociability. In *Letters to His Son* (1774), Lord Chesterfield wrote: "Make yourself absolute master . . . of your temper, and your countenance, so far, at least, as that no visible change do appear in either, whatever you may feel inwardly." An extreme case is the "deadpan," a face which bears no expression.

The distinction between revealing and concealing is another version of the opposition between Lavater and Lichtenberg: the fixed characteristics of the face telling only the truth, while expressiveness, under control of the will, is able to dissemble (10). In response to concerns about deception,

Lavater appealed to the non-malleable features of the face, arguing that these are best captured in the silhouette, "the truest and most faithful image that one can give of a person" (Lyon 262). Alphonse Bertillon agreed that the profile view served to cancel the contingency of expression.

Facial expression may be the sign of an emotion, but, according to Silvan Tomkins, it may merely be a "way of negotiating dangerous or ambivalent situations by means of mimicry or bluffing" (Frow 239). A newer explanation for expressions was the behavioral ecology view of facial displays (BECV) of Alan Fridlund or Carlo Crivelli. In this view, our faces are "social tools" used as leading signs in social negotiation, the way that humans "navigate their social terrain" (Crivelli 392). Tomkins goes even further: our faces do not merely express our affects but define them, since "affect is primarily facial behavior" (I:114).

Or expression may be a mirage: Lev Kuleshov edited a short film in which a shot of the expressionless face of Tsarist matinee idol Ivan Mosjoukine was alternated with various other shots (a plate of soup, a girl in a coffin and a woman on a divan). The film was shown to an audience who believed that the expression on Mosjoukine's face was different each time he appeared, depending on which object had intervened: showing an expression of hunger, grief, or desire, respectively. Vsevolod Pudovkin (who claimed to have been the co-creator of this experiment) described in 1929 how the audience "raved about the acting... the heavy pensiveness of his mood over the forgotten soup, were touched and moved by the deep sorrow with which he looked on the dead child, and noted the lust with which he observed the woman. But we knew that in all three cases the face was exactly the same" ("Kuleshov").

Facials 2

The Mask and the Veil

This enigmatic accessory [the mask] without useful end is more widespread than the lever, the bow, the harpoon or the plough. What are the reasons that have driven people to cover their faces with a second visage, instrument of metamorphosis and ecstasy, of possession by the gods – instrument, as well, of intimidation and of political power?

Roger Callois.

The mask is the moment when the labor of representation has already succumbed to the thriving emptiness of existence.

Mark Cousins.

Levinas insists that one cannot mask the face: "The eyes break through the mask—the language of the eyes, impossible to dissemble" (1991:66). And yet the face is always on the verge of mutating into a mask. The face and the mask should be opposites: the one constantly changing, the other immobile; the one inviting access, the other demanding distance. They may be opposed as voice and silence, as Victor Hugo does in *Les Miserables*: "The Saint-Antoine barricade was the tumult of thunders; the barricade of the Temple was silence. The difference between these two redoubts was the difference between the formidable and the sinister. One seemed a maw; the other a mask."

However, the face itself has often been regarded as a mask; the two objects that should be in opposition are regularly exchanged or confused: in discourse the face and the mask swirl back and forth, into and out of one another: in Yukio Mishima's *Confessions of a Mask*, the narrator says, "At about this time I was beginning to understand vaguely the mechanism of the fact that what people regarded as a pose on my part was actually an expression of my need to assert my real nature, and that it was precisely what people regarded as my true self which was a masquerade" (27). The Greeks used the same word, *prosopon*, to refer to both, and Latin *visus* (face) delivered into

English both the visage and the visor. Mercutio asks for "a case to put my visage in,/A visor for a visor." Nietzsche said that the person of today "couldn't wear a better mask . . . than that of your own face! Who could *recognize* you?;" and Oscar Wilde once asked a friend about Max Beerbohm: "When you are alone with him does he take off his face and reveal his mask?" (*Zarathustra* and Lopate ii). "It was by his own flesh that Gwynplaine was masked! . . . . They had affixed to him a false self . . . . the iron mask is removable; not so the mask of flesh. You are masked for ever by your own flesh—what can be more ingenious?" (Hugo:) (1).

Why a second face? A face other than your own? In ritual and drama, it was to impersonate (and so become) animals, ancestors, demons or gods:

> Masks were powerful objects that embodied the power of rituals. To put on a mask was to transform the bearer of the mask into the totem or deity represented by the mask. Its powers were transformational. While in the modern world, masks generally have as function to hide the identity of its bearer, in traditional society the individual who wears a masks generally gives up his identity in order to embody the being of the mask (Carbone).

The earlier masks represented by their excessiveness a spiritual realm and it seemed as if the mask spoke out of itself rather than relaying the voice behind it. In contemporary horror film villains of an almost superhuman ability--Leatherface (*The Texas Chainsaw Massacre*, 1974), Michael Myers (*Halloween*, 1978), or Jason Voorhees (*Friday the 13th*, 1980)–wear masks which bestow an inhuman appearance. In keeping with their otherworldly authority, masks may also incubate a demonic presence that overwhelms the subject. In the film of *Man Without a Face* by Hiroshi Teshigahara, Dr. Hira tells Okuyama that the mask wants a life of its own, "taking over your body," and destroying Okuyama's morality. He discourses on the "anarchy of the mask."

Marcel Mauss placed the mask at an intermediate stage in an evolutionary arc that moves "from the *personnage*, absorbed within a bounded tribal society to the Latin *persona*, through to the modern self." The route also leads from the *persona* to people who had a right to wear the masks and then to persons as possessor of rights. "The mask cannot be . . . left behind." It can never be "right to think of the self divorced from social masking, emerging unencumbered as a butterfly from a caterpillar of role and a chrysalis of persona" (Coleman). The eighteenth century marked a radical turning point in the significance of the mask. Terry Castle draws on the anthropologies of Mikhail Bakhtin and Roger Caillois and "locates in the seventeenth and especially the eighteenth centuries the desacralization and concomitant secularization of the mask, which was in ancient times bound up with 'the joy of change and reincarnation,' but which came in the wake of the emergence of the modern individual subject to stand for subterfuge and deception" (Schor 94). The decorative mask that appeared toward the end of the nineteenth century had also detached itself from any transcendental function. The west fell in love with this secular mask during its *fin de siècle*. For French writers, particularly, it was the mask of Pierrot the embattled artist/victim speaking masked truth. For Wilde, the truth of masks was the only truth there was.

Historically, we wore masks to provoke fear, to create mystery, to arouse awe; to play a role or to escape from a role (the mask is primal in that sense also, embracing opposed meanings). The mask also afforded its wearer alienation or invisibility, necessary for the criminal, the political protester (the black ski mask of the Zapatistas or the mask of the Occupy Wall Street protests), and the sexual predator. In September 2011, as the Occupy Wall Street encampment at Zuccotti Park swarmed with protesters in Guy Fawkes masks popularized by the hacktivist group Anonymous, the New York City Police Department resurrected an 1845 law that deemed two or more people wearing masks in public illegal, unless a masquerade party was being organized (Blas). In 2012 Montreal passed a law forbidding citizens to cover their faces during public demonstrations.

In eighteenth-century Venice (during carnival primarily), it was easy for men to "slip into the ample cloak of invisibility, to don the three-cornered hat, and to poise the mask in front of one's nose in order to become unseeable and uncontrollable" (Gregor 19). The *medico-dellapesta* or "plague doctor" mask had a long birdlike beak and was worn in the seventeenth century by physicians to protect themselves from the Black Plague. It became, Lynn Yeager writes, one of the enduring visual images from that time, a metaphor for the facelessness of death itself. Women covered their faces in public, sometimes with veils, but also with masks--in Venice, the *moretta*--to keep their pale skin safe from the sun. The Venetian mask was also a device to facilitate proximity to people of very different social status. Gambling men, Beerbohm tells us, wore masks "lest the countenance should betray feeling." Prostitutes wore masks to conceal the signs of syphilis. The Venetian *Moretta*

Muta, the dark mute mask (sixteenth-seventeenth centuries) was worn by women for purposes of seduction.

The mask may, however, reveal rather than conceal–not a complete disguise but, as Richard Brilliant points out, "a manifestation of some aspect of the wearer not otherwise visible," even if only imaginary or delusional (113).

"I have serenely banned myself to that solitary milieu in which reigns the mask–all violence, light and majesty," wrote James Ensor (the first artist one thinks of on the subject of the mask in art); Emile Verhaeren named him "the painter of masks" (Berman 9). His masks depict highly cosmeticized, collapsed faces, covered in a white base (like so many Pierrots), with overpainted and misshapen lips. Ensor started out as an academically trained painter of the bourgeois interior, and then, in a canvas of 1883, the door to a room opens and there enters a little old lady wearing a blind person's dark glasses. Her face is covered by a mask equipped with a long snout and she looks at a man sitting at a table wearing a mask with an even longer nose. "The mask," Ensor explained, "meant to me: freshness of color, extravagant decoration, wild generous gestures, strident expressions, exquisite turbulence" (Brown 12). A singular feature of the mask in Ensor's work is that instead of concealing the wearer's identity or representing an other, it reveals the hidden self, the ugly self, behind it: "I took some pleasure in painting masks . . . . In this way I was able to make a study of the hypocritical, secretive, and selfish faces of the cowardly scoundrels whom I crushed by my progress!" (Ziegler 183).

Masks remained prominent in the modern art of Picasso, Henri Matisse and André Derain. Often they were so-called "primitive" masks, African masks from the Niger-Congo region. In Picasso's "Les Demoiselles d'Avignon," the painting is split between faces and masks: the three figures on the left have Spanish faces, while the two on the right present African mask features. Whitney Chadwick describes how Man Ray's use of masks pointed in two directions (roughly equivalent to Picasso's split): "toward the European tradition of the death mask with its closed eyes and simplified shapes, and toward Modernism's appropriation of the sub-Saharan masks as 'fetish,' embodying human terror in the face of natural forces, mediating between the powers of the living and those of the dead" (317). In perhaps his best-known photograph, Ray juxtaposes the face-as-mask of Kiki de Montparnasse against an African tribal mask.

Wegenstein fancies that all faces require a "cosmetic gaze": "Humans experience their own and others' bodies as incomplete projects that await the intervention of technologies of enhancement, which will help them better approximate their true self or natural potential" (2012:109).

> Poor soul, she walked with painted lips, and wore
> The mask of pleasure on a face of pain (*Padua*)

"Why, with a bottle of hair dye, such as we see advertised in the papers, and a pot of rouge, you'd be as good-looking as I any day, Phoebe," says Mary Elizabeth Braddon's Lady Audley. Cosmetics also provide a mask for the face, as the idioms "putting on a face" or "doing a face" indicate (*OED*). Almost 2000 years ago, Martial wrote of a woman, "You lie stored away in a hundred caskets and your face does not sleep with you," and "Eleanor Rigby" wears "a face that she keeps in a jar by the door" (Carcopino 1940).

Cosmetics had been denounced by Stoics in the fourth century BCE, and this line of abuse was carried on by early Christian theologians like Tertullian, St. Cyprian, St. Ambrose and St. Jerome–or the Tudor politician Brian Tuke ("What shal God say to such in the last Judgement, when they shal appeare thus masked before him with these antifaces: Friends, I know you not, neither do I hold you for my creatures: for these are not the faces that I formed") and the Tudor pamphleteer Philip Stubbes--"Whosoever do colour their faces, or their haire, with any unnaturall colour, they begin to prognosticate of what colour they shal be in hel" (Dolan 230 and Synnott 1993:85).

Hamlet tells Ophelia, "I have heard of your paintings too, well enough. God hath given you one face, and you make yourselves another." Cosmetics have always had a special affinity with women; Luce Irigaray understands the use of make-up and jewelry by woman as an attempt to "compete in the phallic economy" (Anne-Emmanuelle Berger 99).

"Cosmetic culture" understands women's nature as either decorative (created to please man) or debased. Cosmetic manuals proceeded on the presupposition that the female body is something that needs to be fixed, that an unpainted woman's face is defective. Anti-cosmetic invectives, on the other hand, interpreted makeup as simultaneously an index and a literalization of women's physical and moral deformities: "Women were identified with ornament, artifice, and decoration, and . . . their painting themselves was regarded as unnatural devil's work, recapitulating the Fall of man" (Annette

Drew-Bear 20). In treatises on the arts, women's face painting is often viewed as a debased impersonation of men's creativity.

Women should either forego makeup--"Cheerfulness and Contentment," Aemilia Lanyer wrote, "Health . . . Honesty . . . [and] Wisedome," are the cosmetics that must decorate women's faces and their hearts--or have their faces appear to be in a natural state–to conceal her makeup behind her makeup. "If the test of a modest woman was her capacity to blush, the woman who wore rouge wore an artificial blush which camouflaged lost innocence" (Porter 389). Makeup calling attention to itself became an index of sexual abandon. Casanova wrote: "I only wondered at her [his mistress] having used some paint for the face, but it rather pleased me because she had applied it according to the fashion of the ladies of Versailles. The charm of that style consists in the negligence with which the paint is applied. The rouge must not appear natural; it is used to please the eyes which see in it the marks of an intoxication heralding the most amorous fury." A distinction was aggressively maintained between an artificial face and a properly composed one: "This distinction grew, in part, out of the belief at this time that cosmetics could damage and prematurely age skin, an effect particularly undesirable for a bourgeoise, whose beauty was defined in relation to how youthful and clear-skinned she could appear to be" (Kessler 38).

A contrary reading of makeup was offered by Charles Baudelaire in his essay, "In Praise of Cosmetics," and Max Beerbohm wrote "Artifice is the strength of the world, and in that same mask of paint and powder, shadowed with vermeil tinct and most rimly pencilled, is women's strength . . . . Too long has the face been degraded from its rank as a thing of beauty to a mere vulgar index of character or emotion."

The mask is not always a second face--not when it is a life or death mask or a portrait mask made in World War I to "restore" the facially wounded. All portraits are death masks, John Frow writes, since it was the death mask that brought the secular portrait into being, and Roland Barthes doubles this by claiming the same of all photographs. All portraits are masks, "an idealized, fixed version of oneself, to which one is always faced with the task of 'living up'" (Flatley 110). A scene in *Shall We Dance* plays the mask as second face off against the life mask. Fred Astaire looks for his love in a chorus line where every woman is wearing a Ginger Rogers mask. He tries to guess which one is her, and the other dancers tantalize him by removing their masks for a second. Astaire then dances along the line, removing the masks himself, until he does a double take when Rogers is revealed. A common thriller ending, in Orson Welles's *Lady from Shanghai*, for example, takes place in a house of mirrors where the hero attempts to determine which of the many faces of his enemy is the actual one.

"I am well aware that the expression on death-masks is deceptive," Adorno writes,

> While we imagine that the mask reveals the final facial expression of a life, we know that it merely reflects muscular spasms. But Mahler's death-mask, which I first saw at the Centenary Exhibition, is enough to make one doubt such scientific explanations. Other death-masks, too, appear to smile. But in Mahler's face, which seems both imperious and full of a tender suffering, there is a hint of cunning triumph, as if it wished to say: I have fooled you after all (109).

Death masks have long been objects of fascination and adoration, Janus-faced in their appeal, expressing death but also affirming a life once lived–as with Mahler, the power of the personality denies the overwhelming fact of death. Although death masks were common in ancient Rome (wax masks of dead ancestors kept in the home), they entered the Christian world through a curious crossing of face, veil and mask: the Shroud of Turin created when St. Veronica compassionately pressed a cloth against Christ's face and found his true image miraculously imprinted on the material.

No period of history, Ernst Benkard insists, has produced as many death masks as the nineteenth century, which, in the case of the mask of Beethoven or that of an unknown maiden, the "*d'inconnue de la Seine*," became common decorative objects (Belting 80). The *inconnu*, according to legend, was a maiden drowned in the Seine. The widespread fascination of her death mask was the subject of Richard Le Gallienne's tale, "The Worshipper of the Image" (1900), but the roll of tales, passages and references to it embraces many noted writers and artists of the Modern period (Rilke, Ray, Alberto Giacometti and Albert Camus [who compared her to the Mona Lisa], to name only a few–see Saliot for a full record). In the late 1950s her face was used by the Norwegian toymaker Åsmund Laerdal to create "*Resusci Anne*," a life-size doll intended to train students in mouth-to-mouth resuscitation (Alvarez 156). As such, she has been kissed by more than 300 million people.

A singular form of the death mask known through the slang term "deadpan" was a feature of American humor. Of his hero Pudd'nhead Wilson, for example, Twain writes, "The group searched his face with curiosity, with anxiety even, but found no light there, no expression that they could read. They fell away from him as from something uncanny, and went into privacy to discuss him"–and some American silent movie comedians, most notably Buster Keaton. It is the condition of Shrike in Nathanael West's *Miss Lonelyhearts*: "Although his gestures were elaborate, his face was blank. He practiced a trick used much by moving-picture comedians--the dead pan. No matter how fantastic or excited his speech, he never changed his expression. Under the shining white globe of his brow, his features huddled together in a dead, gray triangle" (6).

II

Hugo's Gavroche, "as he sang, was lavish of his pantomime . . . . His face, an inexhaustible repertory of masks, produced grimaces more convulsing and more fantastic than the rents of a cloth torn in a high gale" (*Misérables*). In addition to its transformative and decorative uses, mask in the modern west also references a constructed use of the face. The distinction between the mask and the face is overridden, and the mask is any expression of momentary identity, while the face refers to some absent wholeness. In the modern period, identity is often figured as an endless succession of such masks: "Is there such a phenomenon as the authentic self or I, or is every self rather a multiplicity of facets, roles, and attitudes that is constantly changing, developing, showing, and concealing themselves?" (Grabher 40).

Because of his ontological insecurity, what each person takes to be their true self, R. D. Laing argues, is a mask or a series of masks that they either adopt or have imposed on them by others (Guzlowski). The art historian E. H. Gombrich announced "We have not one face but a thousand different faces" and cited the example of William Orpen who responded to criticism of his portrait of the Archbishop of Canterbury, "I see seven Archbishops; which shall I paint?" (89 and 3).

Denis Diderot criticized the portrait painted by Louis-Michel Van Loo, saying that the artist could not paint him as he really was since he was never the same from moment to moment: "In one day I would have a hundred different faces, depending on what affected me." And the ideas, thoughts, impressions, succeeded each other so quickly that "the painter's eye never sees me the same from one moment to the next" (Bosovic 654). "There is a plethora of possible faces competing for validation as the signature of the self, a network of different possible identities and self-images, in what Walter Benjamin calls the self's 'arsenal of masks'" (Richter 113).

The mask is the name given to the aspects of ourselves we exhibit to the world, the various roles we choose to play. "The face," Agamben writes "is the *simultas*, the being together of the manifold visages constituting it, in which none of the visages is truer than the other. None of the properties and emotions manifest in the face I call 'mine' can be seen as 'essentially identifying or belonging to me'" (90). Proust's Swann describes the many different faces that he sees on Albertine:

> Each of these Albertines was different, as is each appearance of the dancer whose colors, form, character, are transmuted according to the endlessly varied play of a spotlight . . . . The human face is indeed, like the face of the God of some oriental theogony, a whole cluster of faces juxtaposed on different planes so that one dœs not see them all at once (1981:1010-1011).

The play of such masks was prominent in the work of Nietzsche and Rilke, and the concept was adapted by Jung as the *persona* and played a crucial role in his psychology. Nietzsche is one of the nineteenth-century thinkers credited with the discovery of the "plurality of the subject," leading to the concept of the self as a series of masks: "Everything profound loves the mask," he wrote. "Every profound spirit needs a mask; even more, around every profound spirit a mask is continuously growing" (*Beyond*). Rilke plays nice variations on this concept:

> There are people who wear the same face for years; naturally it wears out, it gets dirty, it splits at the folds, it stretches, like gloves one has worn on a journey. These are simple, thrifty people; they do not change their face, they never even have it cleaned. The question of course arises, since they have several faces, what do they do with the others? They store them up. Their children will wear them . . . . Other people put their faces on, one after the other, with uncanny rapidity and wear them out. They are not accustomed to taking care of faces, their last is worn through in a week, has holes, and in many places is thin as paper; and then, little by little, the under layer, the no-face, comes through, and they go about with that (15-6).

Richard Sennett likened the public sphere to a *theatrum mundi*, where one played social roles. Human life was also thought of as a masquerade or "mummer's parade," as Francisco Goya described it: "Face--dress--voice--everything is pretense" (Bray) For Erving Goffman, the mask is the public face we engage to enter society. Any social interaction involves "face-work," the creation of "an image of the self delineated in terms of approved social attributes" and guided by the "traffic rules of social interactions" (12). Similarly, Katherine Ding wrote that the "face has become the image of the self that one crafts and performs in order to appear within the social-political sphere" (719).

Women were felt to have a basic affinity with masking, not only as a consequence of cosmetics, but also visors, wigs, jewels, masks, fans, lace, gauze and "other devices to conceal and tantalize" (Porter 389). Femininity was the most pervasive mask of all, according to psychoanalyst Joan Riviere: "Femininity does not exist, but is only a mask to cover the woman's lack and her desire to appropriate the authority of masculinity" (Sumera 40). As they mutated from household managers into mannequins, Roy Porter wrote,

> Ladies slipped into a femininity worn for the gaze of men (389).

Pierre de Marivaux wrote about a young man who fell in love with a woman because he believed her expression to be natural, only to be shocked to find her practicing these expressions in front of a mirror. For Jung, the persona was "a kind of mask, designed on the one hand to make a definite impression upon others, and on the other to conceal the true nature of the individual." The danger, for Jung, is that people become identified with their personas—the professor with his textbook, the tenor with his voice. The result could be "the shallow, brittle, conformist kind of personality which is 'all persona,' with its excessive concern for 'what people think'" ("Persona").

The face of Harpo Marx

> smiles as it destroys, cries when it is forced to hear others speak, and Gookies when it reads. This face is nothing more than a mask, but a mask that, unlike other comic masks, is a kind of metasemblance, one that is all mask with no presumed person beneath it, only the sheer force of the signifier as empty semblance (Flaig 106).

In a metaphysical spin, writers from Nietzsche on posit masks beneath masks (in a kind of Seussian *mise en abime*)–as French artist Claude Cahun (Lucy

Renée Mathilde Schwob) wrote, "Under this mask, another mask. I will not finish taking off all these faces"--or nothing beneath the mask: "a series of masks, unfolding in a movement *ad infinitum*, a metonymy of faces, like a *matryoshka* doll without a centre" (Sandals and Whiteley 16). Nietzsche believed that the role of the mask in tragedy was to cover other masks, beneath which there was nothing but the abyss, as is the case in Poe's "The Masque of the Red Death" or Jean Lorrain's *Nightmares of an Ether-Drinker*. "How can a man know himself? He is a thing dark and veiled; and if the hare has seven skins, man can slough off seventy times seven and still not be able to say: 'This is really you, this is no longer the outer shell'"–the condition of Harry Haller in *Steppenwolf*:

> But I scarcely had time to recognize myself before the reflection fell to pieces. A second, a third, a tenth, a twentieth figure sprang from it till the whole gigantic mirror was full of nothing but Harrys or bits of him, each of which I saw only for the instant of recognition (Nietzsche 1983:128-9 and Hesse 179).

"A veil may be needful," Hawthorne wrote in his *American Notebooks*, in the mid-1830s, "but never a mask." David Lubin likens the central object in Hawthorne's tale, "The Minister's Black Veil" to the portrait mask, but Hawthorne's veil thins out, desubstantializes the world around it and the person wearing it, while the portrait mask fleshes out and tries to recuperate the original face (2008:11-12). As commonly read, Hawthorne's tale is about the correspondence between the inmost Me and the persona, the face one shows to the world. Reverend Hooper finds it painful to be judged as a saint, knowing his "true" sinful state and has attempted to reconfigure himself so that this inner truth will be clearly expressed. But in donning the veil, the inside and outside disappear--the man himself disappears. The veil masks, but what it substitutes for the face is not a second face but no face, a darkness. J. Hillis Miller says of Hooper's veil that it "interrupts a universal process absolutely necessary to all human society, community, family life, and face-to-face 'interpersonal' relations--the process whereby we interpret faces as the signs of selfhood" (52). Consequently, the veiled Hooper is described as alienated from himself: the congregation "expressing more wonder than if some strange minister were coming to dust the cushions of Mr. Hooper's pulpit;"

> "Are you sure it is our parson?" inquired Goodman Gray of the sexton.

> "Of a certainty it is good Mr. Hooper," replied the sexton.
>
> "I can't really feel as if good Mr. Hooper's face was behind that piece of crape," said the sexton.
>
> "I don't like it,' muttered an old woman, as she hobbled into the meeting-house. "He has changed himself into something awful, only by hiding his face" . . . . they longed for a breath of wind to blow aside the veil, almost believing that a stranger's visage would be discovered.

The veil's career has been broken into two very different phases: an early period when it signified respectability and modesty–a modesty, however, that moved to the rhythms of male sexuality--and a later period when it only stood for the Eastern other and officiated over the clash of civilizations.

The veil existed within the closely coupled folds of modesty and shame (or modesty and sexual stimulation): When Penelope, "shining among women, came near the suitors,/ she stood by the pillar that supported the roof with its joinery,/ holding her shining veil in front of her face, to shield it" but when Tamar moves to seduce Judah, she covers her face so that he "thought her to be a prostitute" (*Genesis*). The veil in history is gendered female: it belonged to women as a sign of their inferior status, their penalty for Eve's sin. By the end of the thirteenth century, women "wore a veil, as was rigorously enforced by the Church; for according to an article of the Council of Salisbury, no priest might hear the confession of an unveiled woman" (Challamel). But it was always a flexible signifier, Kessler tells us: "the veil at times could indicate alternately a woman's status as prostitute, as faithful wife, and as widow" (xxiv). In Sumerian civilization and in Byzantine society, married women had to veil themselves but harlots and slaves could not (Guven 90). According to Gerda Lerner, the veil compartmentalized women according to their sexual status, informing men which women were under protection and which could be approached (Pultar 117).

The veil signified modesty/sexuality even in its Islamic register: the Koran was interpreted as requiring the hair, neck and ears of women to be concealed; they should not show themselves otherwise to anyone except eunuchs and boys too young to perceive a woman's sexuality (Pultar 120).

In a 1647 poem, "The King's Disguise," John Cleveland writes of articles "such as Ladies wear /When they are veiled on purpose to be seen" (*Minor*). The "woman exhibits herself, shows her jewels off in order to better hide her genitals. She is immodest out of modesty, displayed because veiled" (Berger 112). The veil creates a field for voyeurism (a "Scheherezade syndrome"), making women not less but more visible: "The veil, unlike the door, is potentially both open and shut, rendering boundaries transient and porous" (Gilbert 469). The veil that "conceals and inhibits sexuality comes by the same gesture to represent it, both as a metonym of the thing covered and as a metaphor for the system of prohibitions by which sexual desire is enhanced and specified" (Sedgwick 256). The veil is "the hitch in the field of vision that, by getting in the way of what he can see, gets the spectator looking . . . . [it] plays the role of what Lacan calls the *objet a* (or more correctly its imaginary envelope, which Lacan designates as the *semblant*)" (Krips 43).

In European print culture of the eighteenth century, Muslim women were presented as exotic figures, and the veil was central to this exoticism. Postcards depicting Algerian women in various states of undress "transformed the veil and the bodies of Algerian women into visible erotic commodities to be consumed by the French public," anticipating Frantz Fanon's famous contention that "The rape of the Algerian woman in the dream of a European . . . is always preceded by a rending of the veil" (Vivian 124 and Basu 50) (2).

By the end of the nineteenth century the veil had become a primary cultural marker between West and East, between self and other, "a visual interruption in a sea of apparently open faces."

> The veil exists for the West as a fabric and a concept that mediates a number of concerns, not the least of which is the idea that such a small piece of cloth marks a decisive and fundamental separation between Eastern and Western cultures, marking one as regressive and the other as liberal (Grinnell 242).

In order to do this, the West had to scotomize its own long history of the veil.

In the twentieth century, the veil took a strong political turn. The Algerian War marked a crucial moment for this shift, and in Fanon's "Algeria Unveiled" (1965), the veiled woman emerges as a symbol of resistance– "transformed into a technique of camouflage, into a means of struggle": "While the colonial regime remained obsessed with the veil as the symbol of civilizational conquest, women in the Algerian resistance abandoned the veil to be able to better penetrate colonial spaces, and donned the veil to express solidarity (often armed solidarity) against the French colonial regime" (Fanon 15 and Basu 51). During the war, veiled women served as messengers and secretly carried weapons or explosives beneath their coverings. Algerian women unveiled and wore Western clothes in order to infiltrate French urban areas carrying revolvers, grenades, hundreds of false identity cards or bombs: "the unveiled Algerian woman moves like a fish in the Western waters" (Vivian 127-8 and Fanon 80).

The west, particularly after 9/11, reinforced the tension between the face and the veil by attempting to ban the latter. These included a series of French laws forbidding Muslim women to veil their faces and Quebec's Charter of Rights and "burka bans" in the UK and Europe (3).

> The burka practice is seen as a direct denial and criticism of the openness and face-to-face engagement we expect as appropriate and established conduct. The black cloth that obliterates the space where the face should be sends a message of denial, separation and rejection. In effect, the person behind the mask declares (or is obliged to declare) that she is unavailable as a normal public entity (Maley).

"The veil became a screen onto which were projected images of strangeness and fantasies of danger—danger to the fabric of French society and to the future of the republican nation" (Scott 10). For many supporters of the law, the veil was the ultimate symbol of Islam's resistance to modernity (and oppression of women). The veiled Muslim woman represented both the Islamic threat and the creature in need of saving.

Although Muslim women may argue that they wear the veil as an expression of religious conviction, lawmakers insisted that this could not logically be the case, as the veil was an endorsement of submission and an abandonment of individuality.

Joan Scott writes that "the numbers do not explain the attention being paid to veils. In France, just before the law was passed, only 14 percent of Muslim women polled wore the hijab," while Shaista Gohir, chairman of the Muslim Women's Network UK, states that more women have adopted headscarves after the Sept. 11 2000 and July 7, 2005 attacks on the United States and London respectively, in part as a way to "make visible their religious and cultural difference from the West and to show pride in their faith and the community" (Scott 3 and Mansbridge 50).

Discussion of the Islamic veil is dominated by binary thinking whereby the veil invariably signifies oppression or emancipation. There are, however, multiple and complex reasons why women veil: women may choose to do so, Kaya Hayon observes, "to express their modesty or piousness, to resist the hegemony of Western cultural values, or to avoid unwanted male attention in the public sphere." Saba Mahmood argues that veiled Muslim women's submission to religious codes should not be interpreted as a lack of autonomy, but as a means to achieve agency and self-realization (Hayon 336 and 7). "The veil has not lost its potency as a 'visual trope' that, according to Reina Lewis, 'is endlessly repositioned by changing world events and constantly reframed by nuanced shifting responses of veiling communities'" (Toossi 641).

Facials 3

Face to Face--Likeness and (Mis)Recognition

For the minde can backward cast
Upon herself her understanding light;
But she is so corrupt, and so defac't,
As her owne image doth her selfe affright.
Sir John Davies.

. . . the last calamity which has now fallen, and
which has finally severed me from my own face and
nature. This, then, is the last time, short of a miracle,
that Henry Jekyll can think his own thoughts or see
his own face . . . in the glass.
Robert Louis Stevenson.

When we say that someone resembles or does not resemble someone else, we are generally referring to the face: "The face is the point of departure and the point of anchorage" of the entire history of representation. According to Jacques Aumont, all representation is really inaugurated by the desire of man to figure himself as face (15). Because we cannot see our faces–we know the face by touch and we know what it feels like from the inside--we need to acquire our likeness from an image, most often a reflection in a mirror. Portraits belong in this series, as well as shadows and ghosts. E.T.A. Hoffmann's Georg Haberland "acquired the reputation of being an excellent portraitist who could steal likenesses for miniatures right out of mirrors" (250). Likeness is not a simple property of the face; it belongs to representation.

Mirrors not only provide us with our likenesses but also, it is speculated, with our identities, our sense of self. There is no consensus among critics about acquiring a sense of self from the mirror: Herbert Grabes has argued that between the thirteenth and seventeenth centuries the mirror shifted from a figure of divine idealism to a metaphor for human consciousness and originality. At the other end of the spectrum, Deborah Shuger resisted the link between the invention of the glass mirror and the emergence of modern subjectivity. Rayna Kalas added that Shuger "quite rightly observes that the Renaissance mirror was more transitive than reflexive: the mirror was meant to direct the viewer's gaze toward a moral or spiritual lesson rather than back upon the viewer's self" (Charalampous 2). As if in a historical relay of looks, the shop window succeeded the mirror as a site of identity construction in the mid nineteenth-century, and the shop window was displaced by the cinema screen (Friedberg 66).

The formula for subjectivity I have just sketched, however, works only for men. The portrait painter in Henry James' "The Liar" "held that a gentleman should be painted but once in his life--that it was eager and fatuous to be hung up all over the place [as Dorian was]. That was good for women, who made a pretty wall-pattern--but the male face didn't lend itself to decorative repetition" (*London*). The identity transmitted to the woman by the mirror is symbolic; the image she identifies with is a projection of her sin, as in Titian's *Vanity of Earthly Things* (or a superimposition of male desire). As such her reflected image was often replaced by a skeleton (for example, Hans Baldung's *Woman, Snake, Deer and Capreolus* [1528]). In Charlotte Bronte's *Villette* Lucy Snowe looks into a mirror and sees the skull-like image of a dead self ("In this mirror. . . I looked spectral; my eyes larger and more hollow, my hair darker than was natural, by contrast with my thin and ashen face"). Conversely, Virginia Woolf often writes about the horrors of a woman facing a mirror. Her characters and the autobiographical voice "accuse the looking-glass of being a most dreadful device which induces a woman's infinite 'reflections' of self-doubt, pain and humiliation" (Deppman 32) (1).

Alice threatens to push her naughty kitten through the mirror into "Looking-Glass House" where, Alice tells Kitty, "things look the other way . . . . words go the wrong way." She must hold the book up to the mirror to read it and, when she pursues the Red Queen, she must walk in the opposite direction to catch up with her. Wilde (echoing Plato on the duplicity of mirror images in *The Sophist*) called mirrors one of the unpublished crimes of the nineteenth century; Marcus Brown, who was in charge of polishing the 200 inch mirror at Mount Palomar in the 1930s, told his assistants, "Glass won't ever do what you expect. It has as many moods as a movie star" (Stoljar 362 and Smith). Though mirrors are thought to duplicate the face perfectly, they actually alter and distort the image in various ways, certainly by a reversal of left and right and the halving of size; as a result our image of ourselves is not the one that others see. John Tenniel claims that Tweedledum and Tweedledee are twins, but Martin Gardner insists that Carroll intended them to be enantiomorphs: three-dimensional mirror images, mouthing parallel but contrary utterances: "'I know what you're thinking about,' said Tweedledum; 'but it isn't so, nohow' . . . . 'Contrariwise,' continued Tweedledee, 'if it was so, it might be; and if it were so, it would be; but as it isn't, it ain't.'" The most profound alteration in reflection, as Christopher Craft points out, is that the viewing subject returns to himself devoid of presence, returns "only as his own visible alienation, his being-over-there coming back to himself here .... 'a kind of shadow,'" Foucault calls it, 'that gives me my own visibility' by positioning me 'over there where I am not'" (110). Sometimes, the fault lies in the particular mirror, like in the funhouse mirrors in the "Nighttown" episode of *Ulysses*.

Simmel noted that the human face was of unique importance in the fine arts and asked if the face had "certain intrinsic aesthetic qualities that account for its significance as a subject in art?" (Siegel 276). A portrait is a picture whose unique subject matter is a resemblance. James insisted, referring to John Singer Sargent, that "There is no greater work of art than a great portrait," even though his own portraits depersonalize the sitter. Cézanne maintained that the goal of all art is the human face (James, *Picture* and "How").

> The first person who expressed the human features by fitting a mould of plaster upon the face, and then improving it by pouring melted wax into the cast, was Lysistratus of Sicyon . . . . It was he, in fact, who first made it his study to give a faithful likeness; for before his time, artists only thought how to make their portraits as handsome as possible (Pliny in Saliot 64).

Pliny offered another version, of portraiture originating with a maid of Corinth who desired to capture the likeness of her lover before he went into battle by drawing around the shadow cast by his head on the wall of a cave (and her father, Butades of Sicyon, modelled the face in clay), but Leon Battista Alberti used to tell his friends that the inventor of painting was Narcissus: "What else can you call painting but a similar embracing with art of what is presented on the surface of the water in the fountain" (Tudor 36).

Faces, however, were subordinated to bodies for much of art history, or so John Brophy argues in *The Face in Western Art*, and this regime ruled until the Renaissance, until, according to Vasari, Giotto recovered the portrayal of likenesses of living persons (17-18). Earlier, faces were, if not absent, at least overlooked. "Portraiture completed the transition to faciality which released the face from the surface (as on a coin or medal) and turned it toward the viewer" (Belting 120). Portrait painting emerges as a prominent genre with Giotto at about the time the person was beginning to be conceptualized as an individual: cultural theorists have declared that the history of modern self-identity and subjectivity is inseparable from the portrayal of the human face.

According to Charles Saumarez Smith, there are three distinct traditions of portraiture. The first is the painterly tradition, "whereby we recognize a continuing validity in the responsibility of the artist to provide a record of the human face, which is believed to provide an image more long-lasting than a photograph, more thoughtful, more intense, of the personality which is being depicted." The second is the photographic tradition. As for the third:

> The Andy Warhols of the Queen might form the centre point for a meditation on the changing role of portraiture in the late twentieth century; a meditation on issues of fame and the way fame is replicated through the reproductive technology of the glossy magazine. But if one thinks of him more as a master artist in the factory of fame, someone who grasped early that the business of fame had become one of the great obsessions of the late twentieth century, then his work falls much more neatly into place (Charles Smith 55-7).

Robert Sobieszek, on the other hand, divides the tradition of portraiture into a different triad: expressive, blank (Warhol) and fictive (Cindy Sherman) (284).

Basil Hallward tells Dorian, "Every portrait that is painted with feeling is a portrait of the artist, not of the sitter." Moshe Ron describes a fourth stage of portraiture: subjectivization in the *fin de siècle* when portraits come to be understood as autobiographical statements--a "portrait is not a likeness of the other but a reflection of one's desire in the likeness of the other" (233).

Petrarch believed that a portrait that reveals character and disposition is far more beautiful than one which merely copies form and feature, but the aesthetic imperative to capture the inner self took hold only after Romanticism's stress on personality. The painter in Hawthorne's "Prophetic

Pictures" delves so deeply into the interior life of his subjects that he "catches the secret sentiments and passions, and throws them upon the canvas, like sunshine;" even more, what he depicts is what will happen in the future ("Twice"). And for Holgrave, the photographer in *The House of the Seven Gables*, the equation is even more striking in his art: "There is a wonderful insight in Heaven's broad and simple sunshine. While we give it credit only for depicting the merest surface, it actually brings out the secret character with a truth that no painter would ever venture upon, even could he detect it." The painter-narrator of Henry James's "The Liar" "had dreamed for years of producing something which should bear the stamp of the psychologist as well as of the painter, and here at last was his subject." Colonel Capadose's wife, however, tells the painter, "Nothing would induce me to let you pry into me that way!" Dorian's portrait expresses the inner man, as does the portrait of Lady Audley, which gives to the "pretty pouting mouth" a "hard and almost wicked look" and "a strange, sinister light to the deep blue eyes," giving her "something of the aspect of a beautiful fiend."

Warhol demonstrated repeatedly that it was possible to reproduce the appearances of subjects without thinking that it was necessary to plumb their souls. Even earlier, Gertrude Stein had said of Picasso, "The souls of people do not interest him, that is to say for him the reality of life is in the head, the face and the body" and Giacometti complained, "I have enough trouble with the outside without bothering about the inside" (Emrali). Harry Berger Jr. has written extensively against art criticism's easy claim of access to inner truth:

> They do this using an undigested mix of archival evidence, the intuitions of lay psychology, and the record of past beliefs--physiognomy, for example--that often strike even them--the art historians themselves--as quaint, obsolete, bizarre, or merely tedious . . . . At this point I think it is worth pausing to ask whether and why . . . people accepted the opinion of the experts that the face is a totally reliable and authoritative index of the mind, or that the body is necessarily an index of the soul (115).

The internalization protocol, the directive to portray the inner subject, was in tension with a directive to go outward, an idealization protocol. According to Michael Edward Moore, in the Middle Ages idealization preceded likeness:

> In the medieval world, the face did not always serve the purpose of identification . . . . Rather than carefully shaping an artistic

> image so as to conform to the subject of a painting, the reverse was often true: the subject of a portrait hoped to conform herself to the ideal values expressed in the painted image, such as sanctity, piety or generosity ( ).

One of the characters in Edith Wharton's "The Portrait" says of the artist, "Lillo is a genius--that we must all admit . . . but he has an unfortunate temperament. He has been denied the gift--so precious to an artist--of perceiving the ideal. He sees only the defects of his sitters; one might almost fancy that he takes a morbid pleasure in exaggerating their weak points, in painting them on their worst days." The ladies in Gogol's "The Mysterious Portrait" required that "their faces should be such as to cause every one to stare at them with admiration, if not fall in love with them outright."

Photography took over the mission of likeness from the painted portrait. However, Alexander Rodchenko praised the snapshot for being as far from the portrait as you could get; the "unique, finished portrait" had lost its meaning because no image could represent totality (Belting 161). The cinematic portrait is the close-up. For Roland Barthes, Garbo's face at the end of *Queen Christina* "belongs to the moment in cinema when capturing the human face still plunged audiences into the deepest ecstasy" (1972:56). Deleuze announced that "The close-up is the face" and Ingmar Bergman stated that "The possibility of drawing near to the human face is the primary originality and the distinctive quality of the cinema" (Deleuze 1989:87 and 99). Deleuze distinguished between "reflective" and "intensive closeups" (roughly the difference between the portrait and the snapshot): the first, found in Griffith, transmitted a unified emotional signal, while the second signified more chaotically, as in the films of Sergei Eisenstein (Nick Davis 156). The reflective close-up fulfils the internalization mandate of the portrait; it "introduces us to unconscious optics as psychoanalysis does to unconscious impulses" (Benjamin 1999:230). Béla Balázs felt that the close-up was able to photograph the unconscious:

> But the camera moved closer and, behold, within the face it reveals partial physiognomies which betray something different than the total expression had tried to suggest. In vain he knits his brow and flashes his eyes. The camera moves in even closer, isolating his chin, showing him as a coward and weakling. A delicate smile governs the total expression. But nostrils, earlobes and neck have their own face. And shown in isolation, they betray a hidden crudeness, a barely disguised stupidity. In

> such detailed analysis, the "general impression" will not cover up . . . . The camera close-up aims at the uncontrolled small areas of the face–"the invisible face behind the visible" (Marcus 242) (2).

Of course the likeness in the portrait and the mirror are radically different in *Dorian Gray*:

> His eye fell upon the portrait Basil Hallward had painted of him. He started back as if in surprise . . . . The expression looked different. One would have said that there was a touch of cruelty in the mouth . . . . He winced and, taking up from the table an oval glass framed in ivory Cupids . . . glanced hurriedly into its polished depths. No line like that warped his red lips.

But there are differences between them outside the realm of the marvelous: the subjects of portraits are absent, of mirrors necessarily present. In *Vanity Fair*, Thackeray contrasts the mirror's perfect forgetfulness with the insistent memory of the painted portrait (Brink-Roby). Unlike the mirror the portrait was said to reveal what the eye could not possibly see. In John Frankenheimer's *Seconds*, Rock Hudson visits his wife's home and while there looks at a photograph of his old self, with his present image superimposed on what is now both a photograph and a mirror.

Despite their differences, both portraits and mirror reflections have been understood as attempts to overcome separation and death. The art historian Joanna Woodall argues that the underlying motivation for all naturalistic portraiture is the desire to render a subject who may be distant in time, space and spirit, eternally present (Biernoff 680). But they also capture death: in Jean Cocteau's *Orfée*, Heurtebise tells Orpheus, "Mirrors are the doors through which Death comes and goes. Look at yourself in a mirror all your life and you'll see death at work." In Poe's "Oval Portrait," the painting steals the life out of the sitter; the subject of James's "The Liar" has never had his portrait painted because "he was afraid, you know; it was a kind of superstition. He was sure that if anything were done he would die directly afterwards." This duality is held in place by the twofold identity of the likeness as either an immortal soul or a ghost. Like the portrait and the shadow, the mirror image is identified with the soul in many cultures, and "savages," Sir James Fraser tells us, feel that "If it is trampled upon, struck or stabbed, he will feel the injury as if it were done to his person; and if it is detached from him entirely (as he believes that it may be) he will die." In Wharton's "The

Moving Finger" a portrait hovers ambivalently between life and death. The husband of a dead wife exclaims, "How I rejoiced in that picture [of her]! I used to say to her, 'You're my prisoner now–I shall never lose you. If you grew tired of me and left me you'd leave your real self there on the wall!'" But then he realizes that the portrait signifies death not proximate life:

> The idea came to me: "It's the picture that stands between us; the picture that is dead, and not my wife. To sit in this room is to keep watch beside a corpse." As this feeling grew on me the portrait became like a beautiful mausoleum in which she had been buried alive: I could hear her beating against the painted walls and crying to me faintly for help (*Crucial*).

The mirror was easily regarded as a portal through which spirits left the world, and conversely, a gateway through which the dead re-entered; hence the popular superstition advising the covering of mirror surfaces after death in order to prevent the soul of the deceased from emerging to haunt the living.

"I would like," Van Gogh wrote, "to make portraits that, a century later, might appear to the people of that time as apparitions." Both portraits and mirrors are credited with depicting ghost scenes–sites filled with apparitions from the past which threaten to burst out into the present. Writing of the *House of the Seven Gables*, Hawthorne said, "As regards its interior life, a large, dim looking-glass used to hang in one of the rooms, and was fabled to contain within its depths all the shapes that had ever been reflected there." Hawthorne was particularly fond of this trope, for example, in "Old Esther Dudley":

> . . . it was the general belief that Esther could cause the governors of the overthrown dynasty, with the beautiful ladies who had once adorned their festivals, the Indian chiefs who had come up to the province-house to hold council or swear allegiance, the grim provincial warriors, the severe clergymen—in short, all the pageantry of gone days, all the figures that ever swept across the broad-plate of glass in former times,—she could cause the whole to reappear and people the inner world of the mirror with shadows of old life (*Twice*) (3).

"Virtually no Gothic romance is complete," Theodore Ziolkowski writes, "without a . . . similar case of mistaken identity based upon an uncanny resemblance between a portrait and a living figure, whose appearance is first thought to be a walking portrait." In Théophile Gautier's "Coffee Pot,-" one of the oldest of the forefathers steps out of his portrait and unlocks the other frames in the picture gallery, and all the ancestors come out, drink coffee and dance (Ziolkowski 86 and 97).

During the nineteenth century the mirror, on the one hand, pervaded the cities of the West as an icon of bourgeois self-satisfaction; as Jean Baudrillard has noted, the mirror's popularity as home furnishing came from its ability to afford "the self-indulgent bourgeois individual the opportunity to exercise his privileges—to reproduce his own image and reveal his possessions" (22). On the other, it underwent a fantastic expansion at the hands of Romantic writers. Both mirror and portrait were treated as magical, as instruments of ultimate truth (e.g., the skeleton in the woman's mirror) and of clairvoyance or prophecy. In the depths of a mirror one may be able to see far-distant events or the future: the evil queen in "Snow White" uses her mirror for divining. Edmund Spenser's Britomart looks into Merlin's magic mirror ("He who looked into it, saw not himself, but saw there portrayed anything that was happening in any part of the world that might be of consequence to him") and, unable to see herself in it, remembers that it only reflected things that were relevant for the viewer; and so she asks it what husband fortune would give her, sees Sir Artegall and falls instantly in love with him. Angela Carter has her Beauty in "The Tiger's Bride," look into her mirror, "but it was in the midst of one of its magic fits again and I did not see my own face in it but that of my father; at first I thought he smiled at me. Then I saw he was smiling with pure gratification" (167).

In *Alice*, the mirror is a gateway, leading to a new place (4). In *Orfée* the Princess, Cégeste, and Heurtebise exit a room by moving into a large mirror. The ontology of the mirror is such that we do not see it but appear to see through it: "the tain offers a fold 'in' reality, implying a double on the other side of the mirror, opening up an uncanny space of nonbeing" (Andrew Butler 149). Within this conceit (literary here but spectrophobic in ordinary life), traffic is possible, the outside subject can be pulled into the mirror, as in H. P. Lovecraft's "The Trap" ("What was fantasy in the tale of 'Alice' now came to me as a grave and immediate reality. That looking-glass had indeed possessed a malign, abnormal suction. It was more than a mirror—it was a gate; a trap; a link with spatial recesses not meant for the denizens of our visible universe"), or the inside images can burst out, as in China Miéville's "The Tain." The aliens that bring London to a standstill in "The Tain" are, as in Hawthorne and Dickens, an inventory of previous reflections that have been incubating in the mirror's depths. They may have begun their existance as reflections of original subjects but are now aggressive alien agents, simmering in fury: Sometimes when only a part of the face was reflected,

> it was not so bad. One little part of us would momentarily be crushed into the banal shape of your mouth, but we were free beyond those few inches and could gesticulate hatred at you. But when you leaned over the lakes we were pinioned to you, trapped into our mimicry. When you looked into the obsidian you saw, not yourselves, but us, watching, with our loathing (72).

Known as imagos and as tains, they break through the glass to destroy the civilization that called them into being. Miéville borrowed them from Jorge Luis Borges' *Book of Imaginary Beings*, where they were shifting and shining creatures "that nobody had ever caught but that many said they had glimpsed in the depths of mirrors." Kilgore Trout, in Kurt Vonnegut's *Breakfast of Champions*, refers to mirrors as "leaks" and likes to pretend that they are "holes between two universes," which he often warns young children not to get to close to (19) (5).

II

Levinas focuses not on the face but on the "face to face"–a primordial relationship between self and other which takes place, so he says, prior to the intervention of language and society--the basis of ethical humanity and social interaction. Jonathan Cole, an American sociologist, argues that a person's identity is formed through face-to-face exchanges, citing Maurice Merleau-Ponty in the *Primacy of Perception*: "I live in the facial expression of the other, as I feel him living in mine" (179). "Without the impression of ourselves in the face of the other, one lacks the dialectical setting in which languages evolve" (Siegel 108).

Face to face is forbidden when it comes to the divine. "When Moses saw the Burning Bush, he hid his face, afraid to look at God. Later, when he was to receive the Law on the mountain, God first reminded him: 'you cannot see my face, for no one shall see me and live'" (Moore 30). The face of the Christian god is so powerful that it cannot be looked at; hence a prohibition against iconography. This is a trope that is also applied to monstrosity: upon "seeing" the monster, Victor Frankenstein exclaims, "Oh! no mortal could support the horror of that countenance . . . . Never did I behold a vision so horrible as his face, of such loathsome, yet appalling hideousness."

The face is the place of encounter between individuals; even the encounter between the human and the machine is graced with the term "interface." The face is the only part of the body that is authorized to accept the gaze of others; looking at other body parts drifts into regions of pornography. The exchange between one face and another generates a mysterious state called recognition, a spark expressing the information: "I know what that is." We have been fitted with the ability to recognize a staggering variety of faces instantly and to interpret facial expressions as well, an almost instantaneous reaction that can blossom after a mere glimpse. The face is easily recognized, even in the face of its remarkable mobility: "Our recognition of faces is miraculous. We are exposed to so many different faces with so little variation among them. How can we recognize a face we have only seen smiling when we come upon it again while it is crying?" (Daniel Black 13) (6).

Alan Richardson writes that there are "dedicated neural systems not only for recognizing faces (as distinct from recognizing objects generally) but for interpreting facial expressions as well;" and these propensities "occur independently across geographically distant and culturally distinct human populations" (Zunshine 65). Neuroscientists have located a part of the brain, the "fusiform face area," that lights up when we look at faces (Serpell).

In Levinas the face-to-face duo is self and other but within Western discourse it tends to regress to self and self--a doubling or mirror relationship. Levinas tried to break up this solipsistic habit, but in this chapter I will do the opposite: explore how mirror relationships invariably drift in the direction of otherness, of misrecognition. As Jacqueline Rose writes of Jacques Lacan's mirror-stage hypothesis, "The image in which we first recognize ourselves is a misrecognition" (30). The alternative to recognition even has a medical name, prosopagnosia or face-blindness. In a related condition, facial dysmorphia, the subject has a warped perception of the face. Aphanisis (which literally refers to the disappearance of the subject behind the signifier) also refers to a failure to recognize ourselves when faced with a mirror image.

The culture of the nineteenth century abounds in mirror moments, sometimes in front of an actual mirror, sometimes a portrait, sometimes between twins and sometimes with ghosts or shadows or more inexplicable doubles; sometimes between alternates–a young and an older self as in Borges's "The Other"--or other variations, as in James' "The Jolly Corner," between Spencer Brydon as an expatriate dilettante and the ugly capitalist he would have been had he remained in America.

The doppelganger and doubling dance to the rhythms of the most well-worm binary oppositions: outside/inside and life/death. Interpretation is usually divided between a marvellous and a pathological explanation, between the double as a supernatural agent, often a projection of the devil himself (Samuel Scrape tells James Hogg's Robert Wringham that "The devil's often seen gaun sidie for sidie w'ye ... an' they say that he whiles takes your ain shape") and a psychological projection, a Jungian shadow (Gil-Martin "is to be read as a projection of Wringhim's inner state, a hallucinatory delusion who externalizes all of the impulses that Wringhim is repressing") (Thorpe 9). In E. T. A. Hoffman's "The Sandman" it is both: "Now, if we have a mind which is sufficiently firm . . . then will the dark power fail in its attempt to gain a power that shall be a reflection of ourselves" (*Tales*) (7).

This is the first stage in the fragmentation of the self, "a process which marches with ever bolder strides through the discourses and practices of the nineteenth and twentieth centuries"--the doubling of individual characters in order to portray inner conflicts, to depict the tension between the conscious and unconscious mind (Andrew Webber; also see Laurence Porter). Or the overt and repressed sides of a single character: Gil-Martin proclaims that "we are all subjected to two distinct natures in the same person." In the postmodern era, Gordon Slethaug argues in *Doubling and Reversal*, the double is transformed from an alternative self "to an ironic literary device that undermines suggestions of universal harmony, essential duality, psychological wholeness, or stable signification" (Zeitlin). In all the formulations of the double as a projection of a split or fragmented self, the narrative consequence will be misrecognition, as with Jekyll and Hyde. The double is either the person you secretly desire to be (Jack London's "South of the Slot" and David Fincher's *Fight Club*) or the person you secretly fear being ("The Jolly Corner") (8).

The classic interpretation, that of Otto Rank and Freud, views the doppelganger effect as a projection of the subject's narcissism, splitting, over time, into good and bad twins. For Freud, the double is initially "an insurance against the destruction of the ego" and "an energetic denial of the power of death." The mirror image and the shadow promise such immortality becuase of their immateriality and, as a result, are the favored representatives of the soul. This model agrees with the visuals of the Lacanian mirror stage in the imaginary wholeness the mirror offers the infantile viewer.

Rank's doppelganger makes a complete turnabout: "Originally conceived of as a guardian angel, assuring immortal survival to the self, the double eventually appears as precisely the opposite, a reminder of the individual's mortality, indeed, the announcer of death itself;" it appears also as a conscience upbraiding the subject (76). Mladen Dolar understands the mirror image in the same fashion:

> When I recognize myself in the mirror it is already too late. There is a split: I cannot recognize myself and at the same time be one with myself. With the recognition I have already lost what one could call "self- being," the immediate coincidence with myself in my being and jouissance. The mirror double immediately introduces the dimension of castration--the doubling itself already, even in its minimal form, implies castration (1991:12).

Once again, the reflection refuses to coincide with the presence of the model. In Hoffmann's "The Doubles," Deodatus holds his double firmly and, burning with anger, cries, "Indeed, unknown brother, why shouldn't I seem muddled, since I and my ego have just put on another person as if he were another overcoat, one which is too tight here and two wide there, and which still squeezes me." (1969:237).

All that said, I will do my best to avoid getting sucked into the well-worn lair of the doppelganger and the persistence of doubling in nineteenth-century culture. Nevertheless, many acts of doubling are treated as mirror moments, and they are fair game: for example, from Alexandre Dumas's *Man in the Iron Mask*: "And strange enough, too, this man bore so wonderful a resemblance to the king himself, that Louis fancied he was looking at his own face reflected in a mirror." Anne Catherick and Laura Fairlie in Wilkie Collins' *Woman in White* are the "living reflections of one another": "it startled me, as if it had been the sight of my own face in the glass after a long illness." Fyodor Dostoyevsky's Golyadkin mistakes his double for his own reflection in the mirror: "In the doorway of the neighboring room, almost directly behind the counterman's back and facing Mr. Golyadkin, in the doorway which, however, our hero had taken up until then for a mirror, stood . . . not the hero of our tale, but the other Mr. Golyadkin, the new Mr. Golyadkin" (98).

"I hate to be photographed," Edith Wharton wrote to her editor, "because the results are so trying to my vanity; but I would do anything to obliterate the Creole Lady who has been masquerading in the papers under my name" (Pantazzi 201). Catherine in *Wuthering Heights* does not recognize her face in the mirror. Nelly tries to reason with her; but "say what I could, I was incapable of making her comprehend it to be her own." Crossing in front of a mirror, Jane Eyre sees a "strange little figure there gazing at me with a white face and arms specking the gloom, and glittering eyes of fear moving where all else was still, had the effect of a real spirit; I thought it like one of the tiny phantoms, half fairy, half imp . . . [in] Bessie's evening stories." Roquentin, the narrator of Jean-Paul Sartre's *Nausea* wonders if, "other men have as much difficulty in appraising their face?" Looking in the bathroom mirror one day, his gaze is transfixed by an enigmatic, bizarre, even inhuman sight—a "grey thing." "My glance slowly and wearily travels over my forehead, my cheeks: it finds nothing firm, it is stranded . . . . none of it makes sense, there is not even a human expression" (17).

One of the most notorious scenes of recognition/misrecognition occurs in the Marx Brothers' movie, *Duck Soup*. Groucho in nightgown and cap finds Harpo, a spy from neighboring Sylvania, in his bedroom. They chase each other and end up facing off in front of one another, identically dressed. Harpo pretends to be Groucho's reflection, and the two brothers spend three minutes in a mirror charade, Harpo matching every move Groucho makes. The scene collapses when Chico, also disguised as Groucho, enters the scene. But is it a scene of misrecognition? The element of play, of put-on (when Harpo accidentally drops his hat, Groucho picks it up and hands it back to him, a move which Harpo acknowledges with a friendly nod), prevents any determinate conclusion (9).

At the far extreme of misrecognition is the absence of a reflection altogether as in Hoffmann's "A New Years' Eve's Adventure," *The Student of Prague* or a vampire tale such as Guy de Maupassant's "The Horla": "Horror! It was as bright as at midday, but I did not see myself in the glass! It was empty, clear, profound, full of light! But my figure was not reflected in it--and I, I was opposite to it!." Or Bram Stoker's *Dracula*--"This time there could be no error, for the man was close to me, and I could see him over my shoulder. But there was no reflection of him in the mirror! The whole room behind me was displayed; but there was no sign of a man in it, except myself") (10).

Sometimes the subject adores his reflection (Narcissus, the subject in Lacan, the captain in Conrad's "The Secret Sharer") and sometimes he hates it (Poe's "William Wilson," *The Jolly Corner*, Rilke's Malte Brigge or Freud in "The Uncanny"). Narcissus falls in love with his reflection and so does John Milton's Eve: Immediately after her creation, she runs to a "cleer Smooth Lake" and becomes enchanted by a "creature" who looks at her with sympathy and love. She would have been content to fix her desire there had not a divine voice commanded her to shift her gaze and seek out Adam, who, in the context of the culture, is a better mirror--Milton's point being we only truly know our face in the face of the other. In Theocritus' Idyll, vi. 34, Polyphemus views himself in the ocean and is pleased by what he sees:

> I looked into the mere (the mere was calm),
> And goodly seemed my beard, and goodly seemed
> My solitary eye, and, half-revealed,
> My teeth gleamed whiter than the Parian marl.

And Gwendolyn Harlow in *Daniel Deronda*, looking at herself in a mirror, curls her beautiful lips "into a more and more decided smile, till at last she took off her hat, leaned forward and kissed the cold glass which had looked so warm." Angela Carter's Wolf-Alice looks to her reflection as to a playmate, running "her head against her reflected face" (225).

Like Narcissus, the Lacanian subject misrecognizes what he sees in the mirror (even though the subject gains identity from it), but both like what they see. Jekyll welcomes the new face of Hyde that he sees in the mirror as more "express and single, than the imperfect and divided countenance, I had been hitherto accustomed to call mine." But a variant of the adoring Lacanian mirror gaze dominates the culture: when I watch a movie doesn't Mel Gibson or Brad Pitt stand in for me, but in a more perfect state of being? (11).

Not everyone, however, likes what they see. The mirror in Hans Christian Andersen's "The Snow Queen" was designed by a demon to subvert the normal world order: this demon

> had invented a mirror with this peculiarity: that every good and pretty thing reflected in it shrank away to almost nothing. On the other hand, every bad . . . thing stood out and looked its worst. The most beautiful landscapes reflected in it looked like boiled spinach, and the best people became hideous, or else they were upside down and had no bodies. Their faces were distorted beyond recognition, and if they had even one freckle it appeared to spread all over the nose and mouth (*Stories*).

The antique dealer whom Stevenson's Markheim will soon murder suggests a mirror as a gift:

> "A glass," he said hoarsely, and then paused, and repeated it more clearly. "A glass? For Christmas? Surely not?" "And why not?" cried the dealer. "Why not a glass?" Markheim was looking upon him with an indefinable expression. "You ask me why not?" he said. "Why, look here—look in it—look at yourself! Do you like to see it? No! nor I—nor any man . . . . I ask you," said Markheim, "for a Christmas present, and you give me this—this damned reminder of years, and sins and follies—this hand-conscience!" (*Merry*).

Similarly, in Amelie Nothomb's 1998 novel, *Mercure*, a wealthy orphan is rescued from a fire by a man who convinces her that her face has been horribly burned. When she wants proof, he gave her a hand mirror that distorts images. She believes herself to be disfigured and begs him to take her away so that nobody would ever look at her. "Do you particularly like the man?" Dickens' Sydney Carton mutters "at his own image;" "why should you particularly like a man who resembles you? Come on, and have it out in plain words! You hate the fellow." Surveying his image in the mirror, Rilke's Malte recalls, "I stared at this great, terrifying unknown before me, and it seemed to me appalling to be alone with him" (95). Freud feels an intense dislike for the bearded stranger walking towards him in his railway compartment: ". . . on several occasions I have apologized for almost bumping into a large bearded man, only to realize that the large bearded man was myself in a mirror."

The little dwarf in Wilde's "Birthday of the Infanta" sees himself in the mirror for the first time:

> It was a monster, the most grotesque monster he had ever beheld . . . . The little Dwarf frowned, and the monster frowned also . . . . He shouted with amusement, and ran forward, and reached out his hand, and the hand of the monster touched his, and it was as cold as ice . . . . He loathed it, and it made hideous faces at him. What is it? When the truth dawned upon him, he gave a wild cry of despair, and fell sobbing to the ground. So it was he who was misshapen and hunchbacked, foul to look at and grotesque. He himself was the monster. Why had they not left him in the forest, where there was no mirror to tell him how loathsome he was?

Are monsters the distorted reflections of their alters, opening a screen of intense misrecognition between two faces? Victor Frankenstein, after all, describes his creation as "my own vampire, my own spirit let loose from the grave, and forced to destroy all that was dear to me," and the monster himself seems unable to look at his own face: "I had admired the perfect forms of my cottagers ... but how was I terrified, when I viewed myself in a transparent pool! At first I started back, unable to believe that it was indeed I who was reflected in the mirror." Jekyll calls Hyde, "the monstrous [being] . . . that I called out of my own soul." The face that James's Brydon eventually sees is a "monstrous visage" (*Jolly*). For the facially wounded, the mirror scene was traumatic: "The psychological effect on a man who must go through life, an object of horror to himself as well as to others, is beyond description," Fred Albee wrote (Biernoff 2017:72). Mirrors were banned in most of their wards.

Two tales, Joseph Conrad's "The Secret Sharer" and Poe's "William Wilson" (the duplicated consonants in the title should indicate the presence of doubling) offer an exemplary pair exhibiting Lacanian adoration and Freudian contempt. Conrad's tale follows an ironic curve: the inexperienced new captain of a ship, nervous enough about his ability to command, is interrupted by the sudden appearance of a felon and overcome with an illogical sense of their mutual identity. As a result he puts the ship and crew in extreme jeopardy. The narrator claims a mirror relationship with the fugitive British sailor: "It was, in the night, as though I had been faced by my own reflection in the depths of a somber and immense mirror" (12). The double is revealed feet first as if he were upside down (attached to the narrator as his mirror image)--but lacking a face: "He was complete but for the head. A headless corpse!" When he raises his face, the narrator can only dimly make it out.

Wilson dislikes his double, desires to murder him in fact, only to discover that the wounds he inflicts on the other he bears on himself:

> Quickly, wildly, I put my sword's point again and again into his heart. The moment in which I had turned to close the door had been long enough, it seemed, for a great change to come at the far end of the room. A large mirror--a looking glass--or so it seemed to me--now stood where it had not been before. As I walked toward it in terror I saw my own form, all spotted with blood, its face white, advancing to meet me with a weak and uncertain step. So it appeared, I say, but was not. It was my enemy — it was Wilson, who then stood before me in the pains of death. It was Wilson; but now it was my own voice I heard, as he said: "I have lost. Yet from now on you are also dead" (13).

III

"Not to Be Reproduced," a painting by René Magritte, shows a man standing in front of a mirror; the reflection also exhibits him from behind, although a book on the mantelpiece is reflected correctly (with its face forward). The subject and his mirror image are not face to face but face to ass. It is as true of the Christian god as of Moby-Dick: "Thou shalt see my back parts: but my face shall not be seen" (*Exodus*). In the Linder film short, the illusion of mirror reflection is broken when he looks at the other and, instead of seeing a face and a front, sees a rear. Discussing *A Comedy of Errors*, Erin Weinberg makes much of the moment when the twins are not face to face, when Dromio of Ephesus says to his Syracusan counterpart, "A man may break a word with you, sir; and words are but wind; /Ay, and break it in your face, so he break it not behind." The first Dromio sees himself in the third rather than the second person; he has the perspective of Conrad's captain: "On opening the door I had a back view of my very own self looking at a chart."

In spite of this odd metaphoric twist in Shakespeare's comedy, identical twins should offer the clearest example of face to face as self and same/self and other. Twins duplicate mirror scenes (except that there is no reversal of symmetry).

> Methinks you are my glass, and not my brother:
> I see by you I am a sweet-faced youth.

Hillel Schwartz reminds us that Raphael Soyer would sometimes paint his twin brother Moses from his own mirror image.

Twinship is a common site of misrecognition (a third party looking at A and seeing B). In Pierre de Marivaux's *La Méprise*, twin sisters who dress the same are walking in the park. Ergaste makes love to one, thinking he is talking to the other. In the *Comedy of Errors*, citizens look at the four twins with recognizing glances, even as they misidentify them (14).

The Dromios and Antipholuses are not merely twinned, they are exchanged. The play open with the prince declaring that no exchange is possible between Syracuse and Ephesus, but the play is all about accidental exchange:

> It hath in solemn synods been decreed,
> Both by the Syracusans and ourselves,
> To admit no traffic to our adverse towns.

In James' *Sense of the Past*, Ralph Pendrel finds a strange portrait in the London house he inherits, "strange because the figure portrayed shows his back": "His companion on the wall indescribably lived, and yet lived only to cheat him." James has the figure [also named Ralph Pendrel] turn towards him and he sees that the face is his own; the two then trade places. The exchange of twins or doubles is central to Twain's *Prince and the Pauper*, Dickens' *A Tale of Two Cities*--where a worthless life is exchanged for a beloved one--and Dumas' *Corsican Brothers*.

The twinning that should result in a pair of similars often, in the case of women, executes a reversal into good and evil agents, a split that is prominent in motion pictures which blends ease of technological duplication with the need for narrative momentum (in the case of male pairs, as in John Ford's *The Whole Town isTalking*, into meek and aggressive twins). Not good and evil, Lucy Fischer argues, as much as the feminine and masculine possibilities inherent in the female (31-2). In Brian De Palma's *Sisters*, for example, the twins split in this way as a loving and murderous pair, long available from *Swan Lake* as the light and dark Odette and Odile. Robert Siodmak's *Dark Mirror* combines the two most common plots: the inability to deduce which of the twins was the murderer and the scheming of the evil twin to steal the other's beloved. This film string adds yet another formulation for the double as the latent sexuality in an "innocent" subject (15).

In José Saramago's *The Double*, a university professor, Tertuliano Maximo Afonso, watching a movie on video, sees himself in a bit part–"this extraordinary, singular, astonishing, and never-before-seen case of the duplicate man" (167). Obsessed by his find, he researches his other self, Daniel Santa-Clara. Eventually he will fuck Daniel's girlfriend and will have to continue to live as Daniel for the rest of his life. John Woo's *Face/Off* is also about twinning and doubling through an exchange of faces as well as various other kinds of mirror events, all expedited by the magic of movies, where faces can be photoshopped from one set of shoulders to another with ease. Hannibal Lecter in Jonathan Demme's *Silence of the Lamb* takes the face of one of his guards to escape confinement. In the film *Darkman*, the disfigured hero takes the face of a gangster, which soon begins to bubble and melt. In Georges Franju's *Eyes Without a Face* (1960), a renowned plastic surgeon experiments on kidnapped girls in an attempt to transfer their faces to his daughter–a car accident left Christiane's face an open wound. His attempts are all failures ("the irradiation for a 'heterograft' is so heavy that no human can stand it")–an operation which will not be successful until *Seconds* in 1966 or *Face/Off* in 1997 (16).

The replacement face is usually the star face (Rock Hudson in *Seconds*; Humphrey Bogart in Delmer Daves' *Dark Passage*), but in *Face/Off* there has been an exchange of two million-dollar faces, Nicholas Cage and John Travolta. It is also an exchange of hero and villain: Sean Archer (Cage), an ace FBI agent, undergoes a facial exchange with Castor Troy (Travolta), a master criminal. Each principal has several mirror scenes and is revolted by what he sees. When Sean-as-Troy sees Troy's face in the mirror for the first time, he erupts with rage and needs to be tranquilized. Troy-as-Sean responds to his mirror scene with a mix of fascination and repulsion: "Its like looking in the mirror, only . . . not! . . . . When this is over I want you to take this face and burn it" (17). The Franju is an illustrious ancestor of this film; so is Pedro Almadovar's *The Skin I Live In* where a plastic surgeon imprisons the boy who was attracted to his daughter, performs a sex change on him and gives Vicente/Vera the face of his dead wife whose face was horribly burnt in a car accident. She had begun to improve, but when she accidentally saw her image in a mirror she threw herself out of a window.

Genetic engineering promises designer faces. The magic of a new face may be produced through facial transplant (as of August 2018, around 40 face transplants had been performed worldwide; the world's first partial face transplant on a living human was carried out in France in 2005; the world's first full face transplant was completed in Spain in 2010), but more often it is seemingly achieved through plastic surgery or the application of cosmetics. The French artist ORLAN mobilizes plastic surgery as an art form. Her project, "The Reincarnation of Saint-ORLAN,"

> involved a series of nine cosmetic surgery procedures performed over three years in order to transform ORLAN's face into a computer synthesized 'ideal' self-portrait, an amalgamation of features from famous classical paintings and sculptures by male artists (the chin of Botticelli's Venus, the nose of Gérard's Psyche, the lips of Boucher's Europa, the eyes of Fontainebleau School's Diana, and the forehead of Da Vinci's Mona Lisa) (Dolezal) (18).

Facials 4

Broken Faces

I want to live like everybody else. I want to have a wife like everybody else and to take her out on Sundays. I have invented a mask that makes me look like anybody. People will not even turn round in the streets.

Phantom of the Opera.

Whoever has followed the adventures of the image for ten, twenty, or thirty years witnessed the strange obliteration of the human face.

Serge Daney.

The greatest tragedy of the twentieth century, the "death of affect," is now coupled with a "fatiguing of the face."

Robert Sobieszek.

It doesn't have to have a face to be defaced: although it could be a portrait of Henry James (attacked by a militant suffragette, James wrote that he felt "scalped and disfigured"), it could also be a white wall (xxxii). As Ludwig Wittgenstein observed "If I say of a piece of Schubert's that it is melancholy, that is like giving it a face" (Rhie).

The most traditional agent of defacement is of course time. Time does for faces what the ravages of war or the figurative scripting of sin does more quickly. Dorian Gray fears the onslaught of age: "Yes, there would be a day when his face would be wrinkled and wizened, his eyes dim and colourless . . . . The scarlet would pass away from his lips, and the gold steal from his hair . . . . He would become dreadful, hideous, and uncouth." As a common trope in Elizabethan and Jacobean poetry has it, for example, in Shakespeare's sonnet 63,

> Against my love shall be as I am now
> With Time's injurious hand crush'd and o'erworn,
> With lines and wrinkles--

or Francis Davison's,

> Nor all defacing time have power to 'rase,
> The goodly building of that heavenly face (112).

Intelligence is also disfiguring, as Hardy and Wilde indicate: "The beauty here visible would in no long time be ruthlessly over-run by its parasite, thought, which might just as well have fed upon a plainer exterior where there was nothing it could harm;" "But beauty, real beauty, ends where an intellectual expression begins. Intellect is in itself a mode of exaggeration, and destroys the harmony of any face" (*Return* and *Dorian*). Christianity, Nietzsche wrote, "has become a very intellectual religion, with thousands of wrinkles, *arrière-pensées*, and masks on its face" (*Dawn*).

The fragility of the human face stood out in stark relief during the First World War. The incidence of the dead and wounded was enormous, twenty-one million, by one count, and the most traumatic of war's ravages was undoubtedly the twenty thousand disfigured faces. President Georges Clémenceau insisted that five soldiers with face wounds (*gueules cassées*–their slogan was "*sourire quand même*" ["smiling nonetheless"]) sit near the table in the Hall of Mirrors where the German delegates would sign the armistice, as testimony to the cruel stigmata of the war (*Gueules*). "He lay with his profile to me," wrote Enid Bagnold, a volunteer nurse, of a badly wounded patient: "Only he has no profile, as we know a man's. Like an ape, he has only his bumpy forehead and his protruding lips—the nose, the left eye, gone" (Alexander). As one journalist put it, "Not desolate Ypres itself. . . could give more poignant and lasting impression of the ruthlessness of war than this mutilation of the Divine Image" (Lennard 27).

Severe face wounds had usually been fatal in earlier wars, but advances in battlefield medicine (afforded, ironically, by the high number of casualties in this war) and the introduction of the steel helmet (invented in the spring of 1915 by a German lieutenant, shocked by the number of war wounds that battle had produced) meant that many more were saved in WWI. Military technology (large-caliber artillery and its shrapnel, grenades, trench mortars and flamethrowers, etc.), however, far outstripped the medical gains. Facial wounds were mainly the result of machine gun fire: soldiers failed to understand the menace of that new weapon, recalled Albee, "They seemed to think they could pop their heads up over a trench and move quickly enough to dodge the hail of . . . bullets" (Biernoff 2011:666) (1).

Unlike other wounds, these deeply affected the survivor's quality of life. When facially wounded British soldiers were taken on supervised trips to the city, onlookers gawked and sometimes fainted; the men called this the Medusa effect (Lubin 2008:11). In Sidcup, some park benches were painted blue, a code that warned townspeople that any man sitting on one would be painful to view. Suzannah Biernoff has compared the contemporary discourse of facial disfigurement to that of amputation and finds a great discrepancy, specifically, an official refusal to discuss or display faces which, she says, amounts to a "hidden history" of the First World War (666).

In general the broken faces of World War I were transferred to text in Germany, displaced in France and Italy and suppressed in England. A secondary artistic path led to the replacement of the human figure by a doll, mannequin, robot, etc.--figures with bland and empty faces. The reluctance to display these faces can be attributed partly to their challenge to traditional conceptions of beauty. Lessing in his *Laocoon* (1766) had discussed the distaste which deformity excites, "sensations nearly akin to that of disgust": "A mole on the face, a hare-lip, a flattened nose with prominent nostrils, are deformities which offend neither taste, smell, nor touch. Yet the sight of them excites in us something much more nearly resembling disgust than we feel at sight of other malformations, such as a club-foot or a hump on the back."

"The disfigured face is almost entirely absent from British art," Biernoff writes of the period in question. Elizabeth Gumport, in a review of Pat Barker's *Noonday*, added, "It's not just that physical wounds are absent from art; they upset the category entirely." John Singer Sargent painted facially mutilated soldiers but the wounds were hidden under bandages, a facelessness which "is the terrible instance of the presentation of the unrepresentable, a portrait that is not a portrait, a portrayal of something that cannot be portrayed" (Harold Scheizer in Lennard 30). Biernoff allows Francis Bacon to be the exception, "painting his lovers, friends and drinking companions" and laments the absence of work comparable to that of the contemporary German artists of the *Neue Sachlichkeit* (New Objectivity)--Otto Dix, George Grosz, Max Beckmann or Hans Hoerle--who explored the mutilated face and body of the war veteran (667) (2).

There is one other British exception that has paradigmatic force: Jacob Epstein's "Torso in Metal from The Rock Drill, 1915-16" which presents a cyborg figure on a pneumatic drill. It was designed to celebrate machinery's enhancement of human civilization, but the artist, strongly affected by the sight of maimed veterans returning from the battlefield, broke up his sculpture and left only the faceless figure: "I made and mounted a machine-like robot, visored, menacing, and carrying within itself its progeny, protectively ensconced," Epstein wrote. "Here is the armed, sinister figure of today and tomorrow. No humanity, only the terrible Frankenstein's monster we have made ourselves into" (Causey 78) (3).

In Otto Dix's etching "Transplantation," from his 1923-24 series *The War*, the left side of the veteran's face is a mass of scarred flesh with a fold of skin around the gap that exposes his molars. "The Skat Players" (1920) depicts three veterans with damaged bodies and grossly distorted features, and "War Cripples: A Self-Portrait (45% Fit for Service)" (1920) shows four crippled men with "horrendous facial scars" walking down a street (Biro 185). Through their prostheses, Dix "subverts the message conveyed in countless press photos which celebrated Germany's technological advancements. Modern technology proved highly efficient in the production of death and debilitation but could not rebuild the shattered bodies." One, who has a metal jaw, is Dix's bitingly ironic version of the militarized male, in which armor and tissue combine to create a literal "man of steel" (Murray) (4).

Although testimony to disfiguration emerged in the art of the defeated nation, it was not extended to the streets: "According to a 1917 order from the War Ministry in Berlin, all physically maimed veterans were to be discouraged from populating the streets, lest they horrify and provoke the public" (Murray). This was a version of earlier "ugly laws": Frederick V of Denmark's 1708 ruling that no individual with a facial deformity might show himself to a pregnant woman or municipal statutes in the United States, like the 1881 Chicago City Code that outlawed the appearance in public of people who were "diseased, maimed, mutilated, or in any way deformed, so as to be an unsightly or disgusting object shall not therein or thereon expose himself or herself to public view under penalty of one dollar for each offense" (Shaw 192 and "Ugly").

The facial disfiguration of WWI which could not be represented at the time emerged finally in the British novel of the 1990s, becoming visible first in Barker's *Toby's Room* (2007) or the *Regeneration Trilogy* (2012), novels that detail the surgeries and sculptures at Queen Mary's hospital in Sidcup: "'The Rupert Brooke mask is especially popular,' says Kit Neville, whose nose has been blown off" (Lee). Other novels include Jody Shields's

Crimson Portrait (2006) and Louisa Young's *My Dear I Wanted to Tell You* (2011) and *The Heroes' Welcome* (2015).

Disfigured faces had not been a particularly common sight in the visual arts before this time: the French art historian Louis-Paul Fischer noted that "In painting and sculpture, facial deformities caused by mutilations or by the absence of some features (lips, nose, cheekbones …) were, we found, very rare" (Gerhardt 179). What I am offering here is an ancillary hypothesis to the many generalizations that mark this shift from full to broken to absent faces. It is not an exclusive thesis; it also has to be set against a voluminous photographic culture and its circulation of the face as an element of public exchange for purposes of state and commercial control and celebrity fetishism. The erosion and disfigurement of the face may have been at work for some time, but the war offered extraordinary stimulus. As Christopher Townsend states,

> A fractured face in 1923–24 meant something profoundly different from 1912 when in a painting such as Léger's *La Femme en bleu* it had signified the possibility of passage between the subject and the dynamic time and space of modernity that it inhabited. A fractured face in 1923–24 meant something different from 1916, when Pound and Coburn had conjured their first Vortographs, and even from 1918 when the majority of the French public were probably still unaware of what a severe facial wound could look like, even if a hardened soldier like Léger would have been under no illusions by then.

Dix bridges the relationship between facial injuries and the montage cutups of Dada. Disfiguration related to the war, "the representational fragmentation of the human figure, was an essential feature of Dada art and performance," according to Stanton Garner: "The collages of Hannah Höch, Max Ernst, and Raoul Hausmann fragmented the human form with particular emphasis on the face, while the photographic portraits of Man Ray and El Lissitzky employed photomontage and other experimental development techniques to create often unsettling superimpositions, doublings, and facial reconfigurations" (502 and 504). According to Jeanne Willette, Berlin Dada showed the male body under attack, beginning in 1919 with Raoul Hausman's "Spirit of Our Time," which presents the blank face of a wooden head used to hold wigs in a department store, populated by a wooden ruler, typewriter parts, a case for eyeglasses, parts of a watch and a camera, and a telescopic beaker used by soldiers on the front: "Clearly, the head is a soldier, one of those once-beautiful faces, shining with youth, destroyed and redesigned by surgeons."

Brigid Doherty suggests that in "A Victim of Society" (1919) George Grosz "imitates on [Weimar's president, Friedrich] Ebert . . . the reconstructive plastic surgery practiced on wounded World War I soldiers" and that Dada montage in general uses the metaphor of surgery, a procedure designed to mitigate the disfiguring effects of war, "but a technique bound by the nature of its work to repeat, even as it seeks to remedy, disfiguration." Ebert becomes another facially wounded WWI soldier, since, as Raoul Hausmann wrote, "Dada is the proletarian machine gun that mows down the bourgeois Kant just as it does the profiteer Puffke" (78 and 73-4). Tristan Tzara's play, "The Gas Heart," also engages issues of disfigurement:

> As the onstage characters move in relationship to each other, combinations both new and familiar offer themselves to the spectator's imagination: Eye standing next to Nose recalls a normal face, while Eye next to Mouth refigures the face as something fantastic, surreal (Garner 501 and 512).

While Dada's founder, Hugo Ball, wrote in 1917 that "the human countenance has become ugly and outworn" (Sobieszek 201).

"For the Surrealists the Great War resonated as a sort of watershed event that imprinted the modern experiment with a sense of loss and melancholia" (Dalle Vacche 181-2). Louis Aragon and André Breton both worked at the military hospital Val-de-Grâce (which contained a reconstructive surgery museum exhibiting sculptures of deformed human faces) as physicians-in-training, and Amy Lyford demonstrates how they set their art against the "trajectory of recovery" implied by these exhibits (Dean 178) (5). "In surrealism," Angela Dalle Vache writes, "the face is never whole." The faces of Magritte and Dali, she continues, "are usually turned away, effaced, cracked, distorted" (183-4). Faces in Magritte's work are often hidden under a veil, as in "The Central Story," "The Invention of Life" or "The Lovers," which has a couple kissing, their faces covered by cloth sheets. Sébastien Dufay locates Antonin Artaud and Alberto Giacometti in a generation of artists [Henri Michaux, Jean Fautrier, Jean Dubuffet, Willem De Kooning] who reclaim figuration, but with a face "threatened with disintegration, collapse, erasure, an unstable physiognomy that barely exists" (121) (6).

A musician with no eyes, no nose, and no ears is the major character of Guillaume Apollinaire's "What Time Does a Train Leave for Paris?"

(1914), a play written in collaboration with Giorgio De Chirico's brother Alberto Savinio. And it was also in 1914 that dolls and mannequins first made their appearance in De Chirico's art; in a 1917 series ("Il trovatore," "Ettore e Andromaca" and "Il condottiero"), they stand against unidentifiable spectacles or dominate empty squares. Around 1920, Dadaists like Grosz and Rudolf Schlichter began to situate marionettes and puppets in uncanny cityscapes. Carol Poore cites Grosz's "Republican Automatons" (1920) where

> [t]wo faceless, prosthesis-wearing automatons with cylindrical, machinelike limbs appear . . . against a background of rectangular buildings and empty streets. The one on the right is a disabled veteran with amputated arms who is still a stalwart militarist, as his Iron Cross and the slogan "1 2 3 Hurra" emanating from his hollow head indicate (34) (7).

The department store mannequin and the dressmaker's dummy were perfect ready-made stand-ins for the faceless man or woman. As early as 1919, Roberto Longhi discerned in the dummy the modern dehumanization of the body, "a horribly mutilated mankind . . . appears shrieking and snarling on the vast, deserted stages of theatres" (Verschaffel 342). The headless dummy became a major symbol in Max Ernst's work, and Surrealist poet René Crevel wrote an *hommage* to the "great shop-window dummy" in 1933, "modern art's new muse," celebrated in photographs by Umbo, Eugène Atget, Dora Maar and Herbert List (Gascoigne) (8).

Apollinaire was himself a *mutilé de guerre* and the subject, before the war, of a "preliminary portrait" by de Chirico which, mysteriously, depicted signs of future scarring. In his obituary of Apollinaire, Louis Aragon recalled that prophetic "signs prefigured the events of his life; a painter . . . saw on his head the scars of a wound that was yet to appear" (Read 135). Apollinaire later received a shrapnel wound to the head in the precise area indicated by de Chirico's circle.

The face and body's increasing reification or mechanization in visual art refers, beyond the particulars of the war, to the condition of Modernity. The disfigurement and disappearance of the face had begun well before the war and continued long after–in the brutal facial distortions of Egon Schiele, the colors of Matisse or the masks of Picasso. The Impressionists had turned faces into flecks of colored light; within the Cubist idiom the face "fragmented into multiple facets" (Klein 115). "The divided, faceted, sometimes pulverized faces of Pablo Picasso and Georges Braque . . . shatter the facial field and the assumptions of unified identity that have historically informed it" (Welchman) (9).

The New Objectivist's sardonic representation of facial disfigurement was reflected more broadly (and opaquely) in the art and literature of the Modern period. A millennial turn against representation in Germany was given local impetus by the war, but Modern art as a whole, perhaps as a result of the stability of the photographic portrait, had already mounted an attack on the face in painting and sculpture as part of its revolt against figurative likeness. Modern art distorts, disfigures, smashes the face or makes the face vanish; the normal face disappears from art around this time, to be replaced by a ravaged one or no face at all. As John Welchman wrote, "Caught in the contradictions of early–20th-century Modernism, the head/face was either evacuated from the scene of representation, or hyperrationalized (Oskar Schlemmer), or etherealized (Odilon Redon), or radically distorted (Ernst Ludwig Kirchner) . . . . Faces could no longer be naturalistically reassembled and comprehended by any logic of incarnation or 'human essence' or pre-Modern subjectivity."

Dominique Baqué inquires into the reasons for this absence: "Perhaps the explanation is that the art of the 20th century simply ceased to consider the face as self-evident but instead set out either to disfigure it (from Cubism to Francis Bacon, via German Expressionism), or to conquer it, as if faceness could no longer be taken for granted but instead had to be rediscovered, won in a hard-fought struggle." Living in cities, sociologists said, rubs out the face; faces in the modern city begin to resemble one another. Benjamin believed that as capitalism came of age, people lost the integrity of their identity and the human face lost the aura to which early photography had been the last witness. As Norma Desmond declared, "We had *faces* then" (10).

There is ample support for a regime change in the representation of the face around this time. Margaret Werth notices that around 1900, "the face took on new forms, functions, and meanings . . . . Identity, physiognomy, and expression became increasingly ambiguous or opaque in visual modernism, producing unreadable faces and ambivalent gazes." In 1913 Freud had recommended that the face be kept out of psychoanalytic sessions, recommending a therapeutic environment in which the patient reclines on a sofa while the analyst sits behind him out of his sight. Léger polemicized strenuously against faces in art which he rejected as bourgeois cliches (Belting 87). Clement Greenberg told Willem de Kooning that "It is impossible today to paint a face," while Chuck Close said that "the dumbest, most moribund, out-of-date, and shopworn of possible things you could do was to make a portrait" (Hess 40, Sylvester 50 and and Meis) (11).

A key incident in the disappearance of the face was Picasso's portrait of Gertrude Stein--"almost unanimously considered the turning point of modern portraiture" (Klein 111). After dozens of sittings, he realized that he could not paint her face; so, before he left for Spain in 1905, he painted the face out and on his return quickly painted it back in without regard to the sitter, distorting and abstracting the features, basing the new face on the African masks and Iberian sculptures he impressed him while he was away (12).

The concept of abstraction is used to cover so much of the difference in modern art, and it is supported by so many explanations: painting went abstract because it had exhausted itself or died as a result of its own success, because it could not compete with photography; because of a spirit of bohemianism that prompted the subversion of all traditional rules of art; because the Modernist portrait no longer depended on commissions and no longer had to obey the dictates of a patron--and so on. There is nothing literally abstract about Picasso's "Woman with a Cat: Cryptic Portrait of Paul Eluard" which asserts the artist's refusal to reproduce what he sees, as if vision itself were problematic (which it was, according to Martin Jay).

Nineteenth- and twentieth century narratives are well populated by ravaged faces or by bodily landscapes that are claimed to be no face at all. Characters are disfigured by elephantiasis (the Elephant Man ["There stood revealed the most disgusting specimen of humanity that I have ever seen. In the course of my profession I had come upon lamentable deformities of the face . . . but at no time had I met with such a degraded or perverted version of a human being as this lone figure displayed"] or Salman Rushdie's Saleem), smallpox (Nana ["What lay on the pillow was a charnel house, a heap of pus and blood, a shovelful of putrid flesh"]), Treacher Collins syndrome, eczema, scrofula, syphilis (Faulkner's Popeye) and leprosy, among others; by chemicals (Kobo Abe's protagonist in *The Face of Another* ["the leech-like mass . . . swollen and distended, red and black intertwining that it has now become"] and Sam Raimi's *Darkman*); or by fire (Edmond Willowes in Hardy's "Barbara of the House of Grebe," Henry Johnson, Crane's monster, or Freddy Krueger) (Howell 182, "Nana," Kerr 129 and Abe 14).

And you don't have to be disfigured to be disfigured. In Sartre's

Nausea, Roquentin puts his face up to a mirror: "The eyes, nose and mouth disappear, nothing human is left. Brown wrinkles show on each side of the feverish swelled lips, crevices, mole holes." According to D/G, the film close-up reveals the fundamental inhumanity of the face--the face as a "horror story": a "holey surface" that is curiously formless (Deleuze 1987:168 and Rushton 225). Proust described the disorienting experience of the close-up view of the face: the lack of horizon or center, the collapse of figure/ground distinctions and I/you relations—whose effects of magnification and proximity result in vertigo and inhuman facelessness (Werth).

In the following passage from *Notre Dame de Paris*, Hugo is both describing and not describing the face of Quasimodo:

> We will not try to give the reader an idea of that tetrahedral nose, that horseshoe-shaped mouth, that little left eye obscured by a red bushy, bristling eyebrow, while the right eye disappeared entirely beneath an enormous wart, of those teeth in disarray, broken here and there, like the embattled parapet of a fortress; of that callous lip, upon which one of these teeth encroached, like the tusk of an elephant; of that forked chin; and above all, of the expression spread over the whole.

The disfigured face is generally withheld; as with the broken faces of WWI, mutilation should not or cannot be seen. David Lynch's film, *The Elephant Man*, keeps the subject from our gaze, as a shadow or a "tumorous back" (Boyd 1326). The Frankenstein Monster is "a form which I cannot find words to describe." All faces in *Frankenstein* are presentable except for the monster's: "Never did I behold a vision so horrible as his face, of such loathsome, yet appalling hideousness. I shut my eyes involuntarily . . . I dared not again raise my looks upon his face." The monstrously disfigured face of Jéhoël in Barbey d'Aurevilly's *Bewitched* cannot be described: "Jeanne felt a kind of dizziness, a cruel astonishment that hurt as the chill touch of steel might hurt. It was *a feeling without a name*, produced by that face which was also *a thing without a name*" (Thompson 219). Medusa, says Camille Dumoulié, represents that which cannot be represented (Brunel 785).

Writers have a tendency to dissolve the mutilated face into an absence of face–in H. G. Well's *Invisible Man*:

> "You don't understand," he said, "who I am or what I am. I'll show you. By Heaven! I'll show you." Then he put his open

> palm over his face and withdrew it. The centre of his face became a black cavity. "Here," he said . . . . Everyone began to move. They were prepared for scars, disfigurements, tangible horrors, but nothing!

or Crane's "The Monster": "As for the negro . . . he could not live. His body was frightfully seared, but more than that, he now had no face. His face had simply been burned away." And Stevenson writes of Hyde, "And still the figure had no face by which he might know it; even in his dreams, it had no face, or one that baffled him and melted before his eyes . . . . If he could but once set eyes on him, he thought the mystery would lighten and perhaps roll altogether away."

From a commonsense perspective, however, all of these monsters have faces, but not the face that, for example, Deleuze believes in. For him and others, the face is not a biological given, but a semiotic formation, a carapace affixed to (or projected onto) the head. In his essay on the face, Simmel notes that "aesthetically, there is no other part of the body whose wholeness can as easily be destroyed by the disfigurement of only one of its elements," and Michael Cohen asks "If facial expression is impaired or even impossible because of a disfigurement, can we still speak of a face?" (Siegel 103 and Grabher 24). The face makes us human and the loss of face suffered, for example, by veterans was usually regarded as a loss of their humanity. Goffman's foundational study of stigma identified disfigurement as one of its fundamental forms; disfigurement occludes the face to face relationship on which humanity and society are founded. One ceases to register the person; one can only see the damage. In *Noonday*, Elinor, Tonk's medical illustrator, says, "I don't know how to look at them . . . . I don't know what I'm looking at—a man or a wound" (Gumport). "Very severe facial disfigurement was among the injuries for which a veteran was paid full pension . . . . Calculation was made," Biernoff writes, "not on the basis of a loss of function or earning capacity," the thinking being that it compromised one's "sense of self and social existence" (671) (13).

II

Sir Harold Delfo Gilles, one of the pioneers of the developing profession of plastic surgery during WWI, complained that, "Unlike the student of today, who is weaned on small scar excisions and graduates to harelips, we were suddenly asked to produce half a face" (Alexander). All that plastic surgery could offer the war's victims was basic skin and bone grafting. Before Gilles, most surgeons simply stitched the edges of the wounds together, leaving the faces badly disfigured. Jacques Joseph suggested that it was not enough for the doctor to practice "the basic rule of general surgery; he must also be something of an artist, more particularly a sculptor" (Gehrhardt 203). Aesthetic reconstruction was left to a new art of facial prosthetics; this supplement to plastic surgery was anaplastology (rehabilitation of an absent, disfigured or malformed face).

Two sculptors, Francis Derwent Wood and Anna Coleman Ladd, turned their talents to the production of such face masks. Too old to enlist, Wood volunteered in hospital wards, and this exposure led him to open a special clinic in London, the Masks for Facial Disfigurement Department which the soldiers called "The Tin Noses Shop." Ladd moved to France from America in late 1917 with her husband, who had been appointed to direct the Children's Bureau of the American Red Cross in Toulouse. There she was introduced to Wood's medical art and founded the American Red Cross "Studio for Portrait-Masks."

"I endeavour by means of the skill I happen to possess as a sculptor to make a man's face as near as possible to what it looked like before he was wounded," Wood wrote in the *Lancet*: "My cases are generally extreme cases that plastic surgery has, perforce, had to abandon; but . . . the psychological effect is the same. The patient acquires his old self-respect, self assurance, self-reliance . . . . His presence is no longer a source of melancholy to himself nor of sadness to his relatives and friends" (Alexander).

Instead of the conventional rubber masks, Wood's masks were made out of thin galvanized copper. Working on a plaster cast, the sculptor replaced the missing components; the mask was then coated in silver and painted with a portrait of the subject, usually with a "cream-coloured spirit enamel to match Caucasian skin, and topped with varnish to give a complexion." The eyebrows and eyelashes were painted on or made out of "very, very thin metallic foil . . . cut into fine strips, and then tinted and curled and soldered into place" (Friend). "At a slight distance, so harmonious are both the moulding and the tinting, it is impossible to detect the join where the live skin of cheek or nose leaves off and the imitation complexion of the mask begins" (Wood in Lubin 2008:10).

In Hardy's tale, Barbara's husband, who has been badly disfigured in a fire, wears such a portrait mask:

> At first she had not noticed this — there being nothing in its color which would lead a casual observer to think he was looking on anything but a real countenance, but the mask was still retained; and she could now see that it was of special make, of some flexible material like silk, colored so as to represent flesh; it joined naturally to the front hair, and was otherwise cleverly executed (*Group*).

Insofar as the portrait mask gives a face to the faceless, it is the material equivalent of prosopopeia, the figure by which writers lend a face to something inanimate--particularly since, as Satoshi Nishimura points out, the object beneath the mask in Hardy's tale lost the right to be called a "face": what was once called his face is "no longer referred to as such but termed 'this human remnant, this *écorché*' or simply given the pronoun 'it' . . . . its loss is accompanied by the loss of the very word 'face'" (29). Richard Harrow (Jack Huston) also wears such a mask, as a result of his WWI injuries, in the cable series *Boardwalk Empire*.

"The Times reported 'magical results' being achieved 'by the provision of masks . . . which will so far defy detection as to enable the owner to go out into the world again without shrinking'" (Biernoff 677). These portrait masks are both masks and faces: partial life masks complementing what was left of a ravished face (filling out the hills and gullies of warfare). The mask was meant to disappear and leave only the impression of an original face, although this impression would inevitably break down when speech or eating was required. It also maintained a metallic youthfulness as the face around it aged, Katherine Feo observes, while the metal and paint were subject to their own laws of deterioration (23-4). There were many difficulties with the masks and perhaps Juliet Nicolson was right when she wrote that "For most of the wearers, masks were horribly uncomfortable as the tin rubbed against the ravaged face beneath, producing a nearly intolerable sensation" (Gerhhardt 46) (14).

"Nothing on earth would induce me to sit to him!" a woman says of Wharton's George Lillo, "Because--he makes people look so horrid; the way one looks on board ship, or early in the morning, or when one's hair is out of curl and one knows it" (*Portrait*). The aesthetics of idealization do for aging or diseased faces what portrait masks do for war-torn faces; they repair the ravages. In a poem in praise of Joshua Reynolds, Thomas Morrison wrote,

> Thus, great Artist, has thy hand
> To half the high-born beauty of the land
> A permanence ensur'd,
> And from th' attacks of wrinkling age,
> And from the pustule's venom'd rage
> Th' untarnish'd form secur'd . . . .
> Nor does it cease the eye to charm,
> E'en when the real Fair is mouldering in her tomb
> *(Testimonies* 10).

This was echoed by John Ruskin who believed that in "the numbered hairs and mapped wrinkles" of Balthasar Denner, that artist had produced "the lowest and most contemptible art." Amelia Opie described her function as a novelist to be copying "the art of the portrait-painter, who . . . while he throws its [the face's] trivial defects into shadow, brings forward its perfections in the strongest point of view" (Bray 58).

Portrait masks perform such an idealizing function, albeit ironically. Like the ideal self--the "likeness" captured in Lacan's mirror--they advertise the way we will look in Paradise. In a bitter reversal, the face and portrait have the opposite relationship in Wilde's novel; it is the portrait that collects the wrinkles and ravages of time and dissipation while Dorian retains the perfect face. In photography, air-brushing, and in life, cosmetics perform this idealizing function.

In the Hardy tale, the face of the husband transforms from beautiful to disfigured to beautiful and then to disfigured again. "He was, indeed, one of the handsomest men who ever set his lips on a maid's;" so Barbara "wrote to her husband to beg him, now that he was in the land of Art [Europe], to send her his portrait, ever so small, that she might took at it all day and every day, and never for a moment forget his features." After his accident, a Pisan sculptor "informed her that the long-delayed life-sized statue of Mr. Willowes . . . was still in his studio . . . . representing Edmond Willowes in all his original beauty . . . a specimen of manhood almost perfect in every line and contour." Since "the mutilated features of Willowes had disappeared from her mind's eye; this perfect being was really the man she had loved, and not that later pitiable figure." However, Barbara's present husband finds his wife "standing with her arms clasped tightly round the neck of her Edmond, and her mouth on his." So he has the statue defaced: "What the fire had maimed in the original the chisel maimed in the copy. It was a fiendish disfigurement, ruthlessly carried out, and was rendered still more shocking by being tinted to the hues of life."

* * * * * * * * * * * * *

Defacement was a standard way of getting back at an enemy, but, in an ironic turnabout, it could result in new and fascinating figurations. Philip Schwyzer writes about medieval statues which suffered attacks during the Reformation era and asks, "Is defacement something that happened to them along the way, or is it part of what they are?"

> In many cases, the visual impact of these defaced or beheaded figures rivals or exceeds that of figures that were left unharmed . . . . As Michael Taussig (1999) argues, "We could say . . . that the statue barely exists for consciousness and perhaps is nonexistent--until it receives the shock to its being, provided by its defacement issuing forth a hemorrhage of sacred force. With defacement, the statue moves from an excess of invisibility to an excess of visibility" (22-4).

Poets such as Shakespeare, Edmund Spenser, and Michael Drayton would have grown up "worshiping in the company of headless saints" (22-4 And 29). Kathleen Scott, a noted sculptor and the widow of Capt. Robert Falcon Scott of Antarctica fame, declared that "men without noses are very beautiful, like antique marbles" (Alexander).

Facials 5

Beauty/Ugliness

In confronting beauty the soul speaks of it as if it understood it, recognizes and welcomes it and as it were adapts itself to it. But when it encounters the ugly it shrinks back and rejects it and turns away from it and is out of tune and alienated from it.

Samuel Taylor Coleridge. *Principles of Genial Criticism.*

I never heard of "Uglification,"' Alice ventured to say. 'What is it?' The Gryphon lifted up both its paws in surprise. 'Never heard of uglifying!' it exclaimed. 'You know what to beautify is, I suppose?' 'Yes,' said Alice doubtfully: 'it means – to – make – anything – prettier.' 'Well, then,' the Gryphon went on, 'if you don't know what to uglify is, you are a simpleton.'

Lewis Carroll.

The subject of discussion at the Impressionists' Club was a picture, "Circe's Swine," by a young German painter; a grotesque study showing the enchantress among a herd of bestial things, variously diverging from the human type . . . . "They are all errors, these freakish excesses," declared an old painter of the Second Empire. "Triboulet, Quasimodo, Gwynplaine, have no proper place in art. Such art belongs to the Huns and Iroquois, who could only be stirred by laceration and dismemberment."

Willa Cather, "The Portrait."

A second exception to the British ban against depicting faces disfigured in wartime occurred in 1922, in a play by Arthur Pinero, *The Enchanted Cottage*. It pairs a facially scarred war veteran, Oliver Bradford, with an ugly young woman, Laura Pennington, as if female ugliness was the condition that matched wartime disfiguration, and it places both wounded partners in a cottage said to be enchanted, run by a woman thought to be a witch. Through the magic of Mrs. Minnett and the cottage the young people who entered upon a marriage of convenience to protect their battered egos become beautiful and discover a true and deep love for one another. Needless to say, the enchantment is illusory and it is the love that renders them beautiful to one another:

> You love each other; and a man and woman in love have a gift of sight that's not granted to other folk . . . . Keep your love burning . . . and I promise you you'll never be anything to one another but fair and bonny (186).

It is appropriate that their confidante is a British officer blinded in the war. The play emphasizes the reluctance of both the facially wounded veteran and the ugly woman to be seen in public, but they are just as reluctant to be seen after their supposed transformation (1).

George Cukor's *A Woman's Face* (1941) is perhaps the most properly titled Hollywood film ever, since Hollywood's prime mandate since Griffith has been to produce the beautiful woman's face–not Joan Crawford's actual face which is "disfigured" simply because it is ordinary but her celebrity face. After her successful cosmetic surgery, Anna Holm (Crawford) pauses to admire her face in a large hall mirror across from a companion mirror and her beautiful face is caught in a *mis en abime* that goes on forever.

The equation on which the film opens is that ruined beauty is a criminal offense, that the facial disfiguration of a woman is matched with an innate criminal disposition. Anna runs a gang of thieves and blackmailers in Stockholm in 1941. The suggestions of masculinity that had marked Crawford in films like Michael Curtiz's *Mildred Pierce* or Nicholas Ray's *Johnny Guitar* is carried in this film by her activity as a master criminal. She is further unwomaned by the plot arc which directs her to murder a small boy. One side of her face bears the scars of a house fire, and the camera conspires to hide her face from us for most of the film. When the surgeon (Melvyn Douglas) removes her bandages, he declares, defining the woman as a new type of monster, "I now unveil my Galatea or my Frankenstein. If a success, I've created a monster, a beautiful face and no heart" (2).

The face of Cukor's title is produced as a miracle of plastic surgery. The production of the star face as a result of plastic surgery is also the theme of a 1952 film, Terence Fisher's *A Stolen Face*, another film which equates ruined beauty with criminality: "When you tried to convince me that a physical deformity could cause someone to become unbalanced and commit a crime, I thought you were crazy." Philip Ritter (Paul Henreid) gives a female recidivist the face of his beloved (Lizabeth Scott), lost as soon as found because betrothed to another. In this film, however, the new, beautiful face does nothing to curb Lily's thieving ways and her promiscuity.

The face is the most prominent site of both beauty and ugliness, the "chief Theatre, Throne, and center of Beauty, to which all outward array is subservient" (John Downame in Karim-Cooper 30) (3). Ugliness was once given an original role in the constitution of the universe--

> In the beginning there was ugliness–a primordial, precivilized amorphous element, similar to chaos or nature in the raw . . . . Beauty came as a secondary stage, as a result of an apotropaic, sublimatory process intended to stave visceral fears of the primitive formless. "Beauty is not the platonically pure beginning but rather something that originated in the renunciation of what was once feared, which only in the light of this renunciation became the ugly" (Athanassoglou-Kallmyer 33).

"And Adorno projected this equation into the long future, proposing, according to Slavoj Žižek, that the ugly is the archaic life substance that art gentrifies, the force of life against the death imposed by the aesthetic form" (2016: 155). Echoes of this original primacy can be found in the ferocity of the Beast in the first part of the archetypal tales of Beauty and the Beast, with which this chapter will end. Still, the archetype ends with ugliness defeated, tamed, by beauty.

In spite of the mythic originality of ugliness, it began its philosophical career as less than a thing, less than a quality. According to Adorno, it was the mere shadow of beauty (for Franz Rosenkranz, *das Negativschöne*). Both Edmund Burke and Immanuel Kant agreed that ugliness was "a shadow form of the beautiful, its silent, invisible partner" (Gigante 565). It was not allowed to exist in its own right, only as a privation of what should have been. Willa Cather's "The Profile" tells the story of a wife who is badly disfigured on one side of her face but still beautiful in right profile, which she is careful always to show to the world. The marriage survives on condition of the ugliness never being "alluded to by word or look."

Ugliness which began its discursive career as an insubstantial foil to the beautiful--"The pure image of the beautiful arises all the more shining against the dark background of the ugly"--slowly came into its own, however, and was allowed a part to play in the production of art (Rosenkrantz in Krečič 60). Then, in the modern period it came to dominate the aesthetic field:

ugliness moved from non-being to being, from an absence of beauty to an entity on its own.

One of the great obstacles that stood in the path of ugliness's return journey to ontic primacy was a confusion of the ethical and aesthetic realms whereby ugliness became synonymous with evil. As phrased by Lavater, "The morally best, the most beautiful. The morally worst, the most deformed" (Pawlikowska 14). Samuel Richardson's Pamela says of Mr., "It is impossible I should love him; for his vices all ugly him all over, as I may say" (4).

After serving time as the absent half of a binary, ugliness entered into a dialectical relationship with beauty, two poles of equivalent strength. In his preface to *Cromwell*, Hugo wrote, "Christianity leads poetry to the truth. Like it, the modern muse will see that the ugly exists beside the beautiful, the unshapely, beside the graceful . . . . It will ask itself if the narrow and relative sense of the artist should prevail over the infinite, absolute sense of the Creator; if it is for man to correct God? Under the influence of that Christian melancholy and philosophical criticism, poetry will develop a new type and form of art: This type is the grotesque; its new form is comedy."

As expressed by St, Augustine—"For he [Christ] hung ugly, disfigured on the cross, but his ugliness was our beauty"–it testified to the shifting relationship between the two in medieval art (*Prefaces*). As expressed by Richard Lovelace, it was just a witty paradox:

Through foule, we follow faire,
For had the world one face
And Earth been bright as ayre,
We had knowne neither place.

A particular version of beautiful ugliness was presented by James and others in the form of the *jolie laide*, the good-looking ugly woman (Colette and Edith Piaf are famous examples): "She [James's Beldonald Holbein] had been 'had over' on an understanding, and she wasn't playing fair. She had broken the law of her ugliness and had turned beautiful on the hands of her employer."

This turn to ugliness was a return to a medieval obsession with the ugly and the monstrous ("the bizarre marginalia in manuscripts and the grotesqueries such as gargoyles in medieval cathedrals") that had been suppressed in the Renaissance and which had acknowledged the primordial relationship (Jan Ziolkowski 5). Hegel had considered "the representation of suffering, the absolute ugliness of reality" one of the essential traits of medieval painting.

> Ugly, inapposite imagery, considered in relation to a Being so exalted and inaccessible, was deemed a more appropriate and less misleading way of approaching the Godhead than any analogy to beauty, goodness, or truth . . . . The clash between the ugly and the beautiful, between death and rebirth, received perhaps its most powerful (certainly its most celebrated) embodiment in Matthias Grünewald's Isenheim Altarpiece, whose gory, gruesome Crucifixion can only be understood in counterpoint to the mesmerizing incandescent figure of the resurrected Christ (Hamburger 22).

Medieval artists did so, Jan Ziolkowki argues, because it liberated them from the oppressive weight of beauty: "Whereas in descriptions of beauty Chrétien had to adhere to the narrow set of authorized metaphors and similes, in those of ugliness he was free to invent as he wished; the comparisons had not yet been fixed" (5). It allowed medieval poets freedoms that beauty could not; ugliness encouraged individuality of expression when beauty trammelled it.

Ugliness came into its own in the Modern period when all art became ugly or was rooted in the ugliness of modern life. There had been an earlier pattern of aesthetic resonse whereby all new art shocked its audiences and was regarded as ugly, but slowly turned on its axis to become recognizably beautiful. "Tout ce qui est nouveau est laid," Émile Faguet wrote in 1907. "Pollock," Clement Greenberg mused in an exhibition review published in 1945, "is not afraid to look ugly – all profoundly original art looks ugly at first" (Teachout) (5). But if modernity reprised the primordial ontological arrangements, it was because beauty had only been "a kind of defense against the Ugly in its repulsive existence, since . . . what is ugly is ultimately the brutal fact of existence (of the real) as such" (Žižek 1997:21).

The situation in modernity was like the smile freezing on one's face because the beautiful in art was possible only with the ugly as material. Adorno who identified the ugly with the archaic, also noted that the "unjust, barbaric (that is, 'politically ugly') state of the world demands an art able to deal with it" (Pop). The Romantic socialist movement had advanced the motto "Le laid c'est le beau!," and the ugly came to the foreground in the nineteenth century as an independent aesthetic entity in Hugo's "Préface de Cromwell" where he acknowledged the role of the grotesque and the ugly in modern literature as essential components of drama. Deformed individuals such as

Quasimodo are considered heroes of this new art. The modern work resists the harmony of beauty. Modern music unhinged this opposition from its conventional place and reversed the priority; in fiction, the late nineteenth century saw the representation of social misery in naturalist plays and novels (6).

Once established in modernity, a turn against beauty was possible: "The universal beauty which the ancients solemnly laid upon everything, is not without monotony; the same impression repeated again and again may prove fatiguing at last. Sublime upon sublime scarcely presents a contrast, and we need a little rest from everything, even the beautiful. The beautiful has but one type, the ugly has a thousand." The ideal of beauty "magnificent at first, but, as always happens with everything systematic, became in later times false, trivial and conventional" (Hugo). Beauty is boring, beauty is dull. Arthur Danto marked a repudiation of beauty altogether: "Let ugly art do its work without attributing beauty to it [e.g. finding 'beautiful' the worms in a Damien Hirst animal corpse] and also without judging it 'bad' art on the basis of ugliness alone" (Pop 2013:79). Mark Cousins, however, points to another story, "more obscure and obscene, about the relation between the unconscious and ugliness. It is an account of the ecstasy which the unconscious enjoys in all that is dirty, horrifying and disgusting, that is, of ugliness as an unbearable pleasure (1:64)."

The honor roll of texts on this subject invariably include Alexander Baumgarten's *Aesthetika* (1750), Burke's "Philosophical Enquiry into the Origin of Our Ideas of the Sublime and Beautiful" (1757), Kant's *Critique of Judgment* (1790) Franz Rosenkrantz's *Ästhetik des Häßlichen* (1853), Adorno's *Aesthetic Theory* and Mark Cousins, "The Ugly."

Aristotle had observed in the *Poetics* a dialectical relationship between the ugly and the beautiful whereby the ugly in life becomes the beautiful in art: the serpent that causes fear and pain is a source of pleasure when imitated in some other material like wood or clay. The ugly for Kant, and he instances the Furies, diseases and devastations of war, must be reclothed as beautiful or sublime, "for to present the ugly qua ugly would make the viewer turn away in disgust—and hence obviate all aesthetic judgment" (Gigante 577).

If beauty for Aristotle is wholeness and totality (Thomas Aquinas had argued that beauty consisted of splendor and proportion, and integrity; something beautiful had to have all its parts. A hand that was missing a finger was, by definition, ugly) and for others symmetry and harmony, what is ugliness? Defining the ugly was a simple matter of pointing to everything the beautiful was not: as Burke had said: "I imagine [ugliness] to be in all respects the opposite to those qualities which we have laid down for the constituents of beauty." It is, Nina Athanassoglou-Kallmyer writes, "an all-purpose repository for everything that does not quite fit, a marker of mundane reality, the irrational, evil, disorder, dissonance, irregularity, excess, disorder and the marginal" (33). Hence the objections to extreme expressions voiced in Lessing can be understood as a violation of totality, a feeling that the face is no longer under central control: "The large gestures of baroque figures, whose limbs appear to be in danger of breaking off, are repugnant because they disavow what is properly human--the absolute encompassment of each detail by the power of the . . . ego" (Simmel in Siegel 104).

The face of the protagonist, of Théophile Gauthier's "Jettatura," Paul d'Aspremont, lacks totality and harmony (similar to Hyde's "deformity without any nameable deformation"):

> Various features, individually handsome, did not form an agreeable whole. They lacked the mysterious harmony that softens contours and makes them melt one into another. There is a legend of an Italian painter who, seeking to represent the rebellious archangel, composed a face of dissimilar beauties and thus attained an effect of terror far beyond what is possible by the use of horns, arched eyebrows, and unholy grin.

As does John Donne's Floria:

> Marry, and love thy *Flavia*, for shee
> Hath all things, whereby others beauteous bee,
> For, though her eyes be small, her mouth is great;
> Though they be Ivory, yet her teeth be jeat,
> Though they be dimme, yet she is light enough;
> And though her harsh haire fall, her skinne is rough,
> What though her cheeks be yellow, her haire's red . . . .
> These things are beauty's elements; where these
> Meet in one, that one must, as perfect, please.

Diderot argued that in painting, "displacing a facial feature even by as much as a hair [could] make the difference between beauty and disfigurement" (214).

Ugliness, like dirt, is matter out of place, or, as Cousins puts it "an object which is experienced both as being there and as something that should not be there" (1.63). And in fact there is no proper place for the ugly object at all. It's condition is a permanent state of trespass, and it is contagious, consuming the space it occupies. Burke, however, did identify it with a specific space, the body's interior: "The shock of ugliness occurs when the surface is actually cut, opened up, so that the direct insight into the actual depth of the skinless flesh dispels the spiritual, immaterial pseudodepth," and Jela Krečič defined the ugly as "ultimately the inside of a living object (like the depth of Irma's throat from Freud's dream about Irma's injection)" (66).

If the beautiful is the bounded and formed, ugliness represents a violation of boundaries. Cousins defines ugliness as that which perpetually dissolves the boundaries between the self and the other. The repulsive figures of horror art and fiction are characterized by "leaking, unregulated, necrotic, contagious flesh" (Baker 103). In science fiction, for example, the traumatic event of ugliness is the "sudden appearance of stuff, the stuff which threatens to overwhelm and engulf the subject, and to contaminate the subject with its own lack of meaning . . . . the stuff that leaks through its form" (Cousins 2:4). Žižek, drawing on Cousins, understands the ugly as matter out of place, meaning for him "the excess of existence over representation." Ugliness thus designates an object which is in a way "larger than itself" (1997:21). The subject's defense against the ugly, according to Cousins, is an act of vomiting, "a last ditch attempt to expel aspects of the impending ugly object, but at the same time it is already identified with the ugly object in precisely that action of spreading itself about;" the response to Kant's disgusting is itself disgusting (2:4).

"In the idea of men of modern times, however, the grotesque plays an enormous part. It is found everywhere; on the one hand it creates the abnormal and the horrible, on the other the comic and the burlesque" (Hugo). The ugly invokes an extended parsing of synonyms: the monstrous, the hideous, the disgusting, etc. The ugly and the sublime are the most common couple. For Kant, the sublime can be "imaginatively comprehended" while the ugly cannot. Burke also distinguishes the ugly and the sublime. Both inflict pain on the viewer, as opposed to the beautiful object which is designed to excite pleasure, but the pain of the sublime object eventually leads to pleasure: "When danger or pain press too nearly, they are incapable of giving any delight, and are simply terrible; but at certain distances, and with certain modifications, they may be and they are delightful, as we every day experience" (Gigante 575). The grotesque, Gigante warns us, must not be confused with the ugly, but apparently Hugo did just this and allegorized the sublime as the soul, "purified by Christian morality," while the grotesque plays the part of the human beast (7).

Pierre Bourdieu understands ugliness to be an ideological fiction used to enforce the judgements of elite consumers.

There had been strange faces from the beginning: Homer's Thersites, for example, who "was ill-favored beyond all men that came to Ilios. Bandy-legged was he, and lame of one foot, and his two shoulders rounded, arched down upon his chest; and over them his head was warped, and a scanty stubble sprouted on it;" Shakespeare's Bardolph has a face "all bubukles, and whelks, and knobs, and flames a fire, and his lippes blowes at his nose, and it is like a coale of fire, sometimes plew and sometimes red. But his nose is executed, and his fire's out" (Homer 14 and *Henry V*). Among Ned Ward's London Clubs there is a club of Ugly Faces: "Notable members included a man with 'a chin as long as a grave patriarchal beard … in a shape like a shoeing horn,' another 'with a disfigured mouth like a gallon pot,' and one individual who had 'a pair of convex cheeks, as if, Aeolus, the god of the winds, had stopped his breath for a time'" (Woods 147).

Of the various male categories mantled in ugliness, the class of philosophers is primary. Socrates was ugly and "spoke about loving the ugly;" Aesop was deformed (Gigante 587). Moses Mendelssohn, "famous not only for being a wise Jew, but an ugly one; as a hunchback, his body was stunted and short, and he had a prominent nose and thick lips. He seemed to embody philosophical morality, religious irrationality, and physical ugliness" (Hochman 3).

As a cultural marker, ugliness in men usually connotes a villainous nature. Ugliness, however, has generally been inflected as feminine in Western culture. Women are most often disfigured by nature (or the biases of a patriarchal culture) into a condition called ugliness, when they are no longer sexual lures or capable of being mothers. For all of human history, beauty has exerted a ruthless tyranny over the fates of women (and men), determining who could lead lives of satisfaction and content and who was condemned to misery, projecting immoral characteristics onto the object that it labeled as ugly. Beauty is a masculine construct, imposed on a "naturally" ugly female body. Sara Rodrigues and Ela Przybylo insist that we understand ugliness not as an aesthetic but as a politics. Ugliness is a category that "demarcates ones rights and access to social, cultural and political spaces. What we look like functions as a key determinant in what kind of life we can expect to live" (1).

Medusa, the exemplar of the hideous woman, is deeply involved in the dialectic of beauty and ugliness. Like the loathly lady of medieval literature, Medusa had mutated from a very different condition. Originally a ravishingly beautiful maiden, "the jealous aspiration of many suitors," she had boasted that she was more beautiful than Athena; so the goddess punished her by transforming her face into the Gorgon's head. Athena and Medusa circle one another in a dance of beauty and ugliness. Athena invented the flute in order to imitate the hissing of the snakes on Medusa's head as she was being decapitated. However, she had to give up playing the flute because it distorted her face (i.e., transformed her into Medusa). The faces of Athena and Medusa are on opposite sides of Athena's aegis, Beth Seelig observes: Athena hid her face behind the shield to avoid see the rape of Medusa, and later Medusa's face is inscribed on the aegis to frighten enemies with a declaration of the female power she had appropriated from the vanquished goddess (899-900).

But Medusa's head, if we follow Freud, is the pudendum writ upwards. Is it ugly or beautiful? Medusa is a "dame" with a "face between her forks" (*Lear*). Like the old Greek nurse, Baubo [a name for the dildo], she is an example of the woman as pudendum. Baubo had cheered up a mourning Demeter by pulling up her dress and making Demeter laugh, and she is usually depicted as a face above a vulva with two chubby legs. But according to Stephen Wilk, Medusa's head is an aestheticized portrayal of the human face one to two weeks after death when gases from putrefaction cause the body to bloat, pushing out the eyes and tongue (de Fren 243). Baubo images can be found in René Magritte's "Le Viol" and Céline Sciamma's "Portrait of a Lady on Fire": when the artist, Marianne, draws her self-portrait, she is looking at Héloïse's naked body stretched out on a bed, but looking particularly at a small mirror placed in front of Héloïse's pubis (see also Bonfante).

> She was the ugliest living thing he had ever set eyes on. Her nose was like a pig's snout, from a misshapen mouth stuck out two yellowing rows of horse's teeth; her cheeks were covered in sores; she had only one eye, rheumy and red-rimmed, and from a naked scalp hung a few lank strands. of hair (*Sir*).

The dialectic of beauty and ugliness is the ostensible subject of the archetypal tales of Beauty and the Beast (or Cupid and Psyche, the Frog

Prince, the Ugly Duckling, etc.) (8). In many versions, the beautiful maiden must learn to love the beast for all his repellant ugliness; in others it is a man who must agree to wed or bed the hag. This narrative arc is played backwards in tales like Hawthorne's "Mrs. Bullfrog" (also a familiar joke), where a beautiful woman turns into a grotesque just before getting into bed, removing her false hair, false teeth, etc.: "The most awful circumstance of the affair is yet to be told; for this ogre, or whatever it was, had a riding-habit like Mrs. Bullfrog's, and also a green silk calash. In my terror and turmoil of mind, I could imagine nothing less, than that the Old Nick, at the moment of our overturn, had annihilated my wife and jumped into her petticoats" (*Mosses*) (9).

How do you live with ugliness, how do you love a monster? "Beauty and the Beast" and the Arthurian tales of the "loathly lady" all address the problem. However, they signally fail to answer it, since the monster is very quickly transformed into the most handsome man (or the most beautiful woman) the subject has ever seen, as if imitating the series of illustrations in Lavater's *Essays on Physiognomy*, detailing the 24 steps needed to transform a frog into the Apollo Belvedere. "Beauty and the Beast" should be the central node of this dialectic, but instead it's a ruse. "The Ugly Duckling" is even more glib: the subject was a beauty all along, appearing to be ugly only because of a misclassification. Furthermore, "Beauty and the Beast" occludes the dialectic of beauty and ugliness in the sense that beauty is as extreme, as monstrous, in the female as bestiality is in the male (or, as Salman Rushdie writes in *Shame*, "what if a Beastji somehow lurked inside Beauty Bibi?") (163).

Is the ease of the transformation, of the solution of the conflict between beauty and ugliness in these tales offset by some allegorical validity in the tales? What is glib on the narrative surface may have sufficient allegorical heft to redeem it. Dennis DeNitto reads the monstrous male presence in the archetype as a projection of male sexuality (as are the bestial avatars of Jove awooing or the wolf in "Little Red Riding Hood"), and the tale as about a virgin coming to terms with that sexuality: "The transformation of the beast into a handsome prince is simply a printout of the phrase 'falling in love'" (136). Such an interpretation makes the ugliness a projection of timidity. Similarly the frog in "Frog Prince" tales is said to represent simultaneously the "treasure" of consummated sexuality and, for the Princess, an obstacle (its unknown or loathesome qualities) to acceptance of the treasure.

Facials 6

The Smile and the Scream, etc

Antiquity keeps the mouth almost closed,
even though the head expresses a scream.
Franz Christoph van Scheyb.

Déruchette possessed this smile: we may even say that this smile was Déruchette herself. There is one thing which has more resemblance to ourselves than even our face, and that is our expression: but there is yet another thing which more resembles us than this, and that is our smile.
Hugo, *Toilers of the Sea.*

Francis [Bacon] was fascinated by extreme forms of facial expression and the mouth stretched open to full gape was his favourite. One day he amused me by saying, in an apologetic tone: "You know, I think I've got the scream, but I am having terrible trouble with the smile."
Desmond Morris.

The mouth is the most mobile of the facial features, an "orifice of respiration, the den where the pact of a kiss is sealed . . . an oily factory of mastication" (Michel Leiris in Kahn 300). In Georges Bataille's "The Lugubrious Game," the Marquis de Sade explains that "The mouth is the beginning or, if one prefers, the prow of animals; in the most characteristic cases, it is the most living part, in other words, the most terrifying for neighboring animals." Historically the mouth has been associated with animals and with the female body or the feminized male body, but one institution privileges the mouth over other organs of perception: the Eucharist (Kaiser 30). And on other important occasions, human life is concentrated in the mouth: fury makes men grind their teeth, terror and atrocious suffering transform the mouth into an organ of screams.

Christina Rossetti's "Goblin Market" has a character known as "Mouth Boy" who has arms, legs, a head, like ordinary people, but his face exhibits only one feature, a wide mouth. When Mrs. Hall catches a glimpse of H. G. Wells's Invisible Man she has the impression of an "enormous mouth wide open—a vast and incredible mouth that swallowed the whole of the lower portion of his face." Like Shiva's half-lion, the mouth in Bruce Nauman's art is transfigured into a self-devouring mechanism that ingests the living body from inside out in the neon anagram Eat Death of 1972 and the Anthro/Socio of 1991, a complex video installation chanting repeatedly "Feed me/Eat me/Anthropology" (Marcoci 12).

The gaping mouth is a familiar figure in grotesque art; often an entrance to hell, For Mikhail Bakhtin, the mouth's association with swallowing gestures at a "bodily underworld" (325). Emile Mâle states that "almost all thirteenth-century representations of the Last Judgment show an enormous mouth vomiting flames, into which the damned are thrown," and in bodily topography hell is represented as Lucifer's gaping jaws: the fifteenth century illustration of hell from *The Book of Hours of Catherine of Cleves,* shows "the threat of being swallowed up and digested by mouths inside mouths" (Mâle 379 and O'Bryan 113). The Orsini "Hell Mouth" in the *Sacro Bosco* (sacred grove) in Bomarzo, Northern Italy, recalls, Luke Morgan tells us,

> a wide range of traditions . . . . Its sources include the satanic jaws of hell of Anglo-Saxon imagery, the gaping mouths of northern European antipapal propaganda, the boccaccione of the Roman carnival, the grotesque masks of ancient and postclassical architecture and the prophetic Bocca Della Verita [Mouth of Truth, in Rome] (98).

Open mouths and lolling tongues were, for John Ruskin, the marks of the "the ignoble grotesque" (*Stones*) (1).

The mouth is the site at which the self merges physically with the world outside its corporeal boundaries, the gateway through which foreign objects enter the body. It is also the passage to the pulmonary and the digestive systems as well as an exit from these two systems for both for carbon dioxide and more pathological forms of expulsion, such as coughing, vomiting, or bleeding from the mouth.

The mouth into which food and drink go is balanced by the mouth out of which come speech and song. Jean-Luc Nancy opposes the mouth to the face as an alternate foundation for theorizing and an ethical frontier. Whereas Levinas's ethic of the face offers loving in exchange for killing, Nancy's ethic of the mouth can make no such offer: you eat what you love.

The mouth can only admonish you to eat well. There are two mouths in Nancy, *bucca* (an "eating-speaking-breathing-spitting, incorporation and introjection, contraction and distension" site) and *os* (the mouth of orality) (Guyer 90). Bucca is a more primordial mouth, one that "gapes open ready to scream, to eat or swallow;" "a mouth that open and closes around the breast and an ethics prior to any face" (Chatzopoulos). See also Agamben's distinction between the open and the closed mouth, the animal world of "bha" versus the human world of "mu"–"in the fairy tale, man is struck dumb, and animals emerge from the pure language of nature in order to speak" (1993:61). The opposition that Agamben registers is a version of the opposition between two notions of nonsense, the nonsenses of surface and depth, "the open play of surfaces and the sealed closure of terrible, inaccessible depths--that Deleuze discovers in his analysis of Carroll." Deleuze identifies two modes of nonsense, distinguishing between a literature of the face and a literature of the mouth: "On the one hand, he describes a nonsense of face and figure, which he associates with Carroll's punning and play; on the other hand, he demarcates a nonsense of depth and orifices, which he associates with Artaud's snapping, grinding, grasping and swallowing" (Guyer 820).

The mouth is also the basis of a new realm of aesthetic judgment that emerged in the eighteenth century, insofar as it was governed by the metaphorics of taste. An entry by Voltaire for the 1778 *Encyclopédie* made the connection explicit: "this gift for distinguishing our foods has produced in all known languages the metaphor that uses the word taste to express sensitivity to the beauty and defects of all arts" (Vercelloni 10). The aesthetic metaphor came out of an earlier distinction between higher and lower senses of taste-- one requiring distance from the object, the other proximity and immediacy (2).

Taste had to be detached from the sin of gluttony; it had to shift from a word that referred to eating in general to the eating of more delicate, refined foods (the polite *bon goût*)–"displacing the organ of taste from the shameful lower cavities of the body--the gullet and stomach--up to a more noble part of the mouth: the palate" (Von Hoffmann 138). Sensibility had to move from swallowing to taste: "A disembodied mouth, a spectral orality, haunts the concept of taste . . . . The eighteenth-century Man of Taste, the discriminating *Homo sapiens*, governs his rumbling stomach with his sensitive tongue, pitting his mouth against itself, just as an expert wine taster demonstrates her superior powers of appreciation by refusing to swallow the vintage she samples" (Kaiser 48). Michel Chaouli speculates that Kant's insistence on exiling the disgusting from aesthetic consideration stemmed from "his persistent worry that there might be a slippage between taste, the agency of aesthetic judgment, and taste, the organic sense" (127).

In 1787, Elizabeth Vigée-Lebrun displayed a self-portrait with her daughter: the artist is smiling. Although there is little about this pose that seems in any way exceptional to us, exception was "furiously taken"--

> "An affectation which artists, art-lovers and persons of taste have been united in condemning," wrote an anonymous commentator, "and which finds no precedent amongst the Ancients, is that in smiling she shows her teeth. This affectation is particularly out of place in a mother" (Colin Jones 1).

The mouth was always problematic from an aesthetic perspective because it exposed the body's interior. The smile in portraiture belonged then mainly to dementia and other forms of madness.

By 1789, however, the smile had been redeemed, the earlier smile replaced by a Parisian smile of sensibility:

> A new facial regime, a new regime of faciality, and what we can recognise as the new, modern smile, was in gestation . . . . The smile was not--as in the crushingly monotonous court culture still being performed out at Versailles--an insincere, artificial and tight-lipped grimace aimed at hiding true feelings or acting out repressed aggression. Rather, it offered a transparent pathway into the soul.

"In the new literature of sensibility by Richardson and Rousseau [aided by improvements in dental technology], smiles were 'enchanting,' 'sweet,' 'agreeable,' 'friendly' and 'virtuous'" (Colin Jones 11 and 15).

Extreme expressions, however, were still governed by the strictures in *Laocoön*:

> There are passions and degrees of passion whose expression produces the most hideous contortions of the face . . . . These passions the old artists either refrained altogether from representing, or softened into emotions which were capable of being expressed with some degree of beauty. The simple opening of the mouth, apart from the violent and repulsive contortions it causes in the other parts of the face, is a blot on a painting; and a cavity in a statue is productive of the worst possible effect.

One salient exception was the character heads of Franz Xaver Messerschmidt (1736-83), the German-Austrian sculptor, who produced a notorious collection of busts with faces contorted into extreme expressions in an attempt to set down the sixty-four variations on the grimaces of the human face. Another is the protagonist Gwynplaine of Hugo's *The Man Who Laughs*. The heroine of the novel is blind and like a typical blind lover she confirms the identity and beauty of her beloved by feeling his face. She determines that he is happy--because he is smiling. She is wrong because that smile is a permanent rictus sculpted onto his face--"The laugh which he had not placed, himself, on his brow, on his eyelids, on his mouth, he could not remove. It had been stamped for ever on his face. It was automatic, and the more irresistible because it seemed petrified"--a hideous malformation inflicted on him by a band of wanderers called "*Comprachicos*," criminals who mutilate and disfigure children. The *comprachico* surgeon

> had enlarged the mouth, cut away the lips, laid bare the gums, distended the ears, cut the cartilages, displaced the eyelids and the cheeks, enlarged the zygomatic muscle, pressed the scars and cicatrices to a level, turned back the skin over the lesions whilst the face was distorted...[all] of which resulted in that wonderful and appalling work of art, the mask which Gwynplaine wore (3).

In *Notre Dame de Paris*, Quasimodo is first seen at a grimacing contest ("eyelids turned up to the reds, a mouth open like a maw, and a brow wrinkled like our hussar boots of the Empire"), which he wins to become Prince of Fools:

> That was, in fact, a marvelous grimace which was beaming at that moment through the aperture in the rose window . . . . The acclamation was unanimous; people rushed towards the chapel. They made the lucky Pope of the Fools come forth in triumph. But it was then that surprise and admiration attained their highest pitch; the grimace was his face (4).

Batman's nemesis, the Joker, also marked with a rictus, is said to have been based on Gwynplaine–particularly Conrad Veidt's portrayal in a 1928 silent film. The Joker also leaves his victims with grins on *their* faces, an effect of Smilex Gas: "As my plastic surgeon always said, if you've gotta go, go with a smile!" (Rodriguez). Both Gwynplaine and the Joker possess a Cheshire grin (also known as a Glasgow smile), caused by a cut from the corners of a victim's mouth to the ears, leaving a scar in the shape of a smile (5). And Gwynplaine's grin bears a distant family resemblance to the smile of Lewis Carroll's Cheshire cat, which grins from ear to ear, and his alligator:

> How cheerfully he seems to grin,
> How neatly spreads his claws,
> And welcomes little fishes in,
> With gently smiling jaws.

Or Moby Dick himself: "So, call him the Hyena Whale, if you please. His voracity is well known, and from the circumstance that the inner angles of his lips are curved upwards, he carries an everlasting Mephistophelean grin on his face."

The cat's smile is like the smile of Reverend Hooper in Hawthorne's tale of the black veil—"A sad smile gleamed faintly from beneath the black veil, and flickered about his mouth, glimmering as he disappeared"--or the man in Bacon's *Painting* of 1946–"already a disquieting and disappearing smile in the head of the man underneath the umbrella"--or his 1954 Pope—"one senses that the smile will survive the effacement of the body;" and it remains after the animal itself has disappeared (Hawthorne, *Twice* and Deleuze 2002:21 and 28).

Although the smile came late to representation because of the unsightliness of teeth before the fluoride revolution in the mid-twentieth century, it became a prime marker of capitalism, one of the select drivers of that system: the sign of emotional labor or forced cheer. The smile that was discouraged in the painterly tradition took over Western culture. "The Great American Smile" smiles down at us from every billboard and every political campaign poster; the happy face is stamped on almost every artifact in the capitalist economy, from Band-Aids to diapers. Prostitutes fake orgasms, nurses comfort the sick, flight attendants calm nervous fliers. Mick Kelly in Carson McCullers' *The Heart is a Lonely Hunter* works in Costume Jewelry: "It was the small of her back and her face that got so tired. Their motto was supposed to be 'Keep on your toes and smile.' Once she was out of the store she had to frown a long time to get her face natural again." The smile of moral uplift is also what popular song urges, songs like "Pack Up your Troubles," "Put on a Happy Face" or "Get Happy."

In 1911, the songbook for the United Commercial Travellers fraternal association had these lyrics:

I smile because I know it pays.
It means dollars and cents in many ways ....
I can't sell goods with a hard luck tale,
So I smile, keep happy, and make my sale (Strasser 168).

By 1920, businesses acknowledged their management of employees' faces: "That year, an advertisement by the Goldenbaum & Morgan menswear store in Trenton, NJ, bragged that they had 'salesmen who have been taught to smile whether they like it or not'" (Brisini 10). At the food chain Pret À Manger, employees are required to be enthusiastic, genuinely friendly and happy to be themselves. But an ad for El Al airlines queried "Maybe You Don't Want to Look at a Painted-on Smile All the Way to Europe," showing a stewardness with the black line of her smile extending to mid cheek. Smiles were taught, by, among others, Professor Palmari in his "school for smiles": "For a fee, the Professor would study and analyze a student's grin, calculate its angles, offer lessons and alterations--even going so far as to introduce mechanical devices called 'smile casts' into the student's mouth" (Brisini 1).

Blackface minstrels (and their enslaved originals) put on a happy face. The happy face was designed in 1963 by Harvey Ball who was hired to create a logo to improve customer service and employee cooperation for the State Mutual Life Assurance Company of America. Emojis, derived from the visual style of Japanese manga, started as buttons sporting a smiling face (a yellow circle with two black dots for eyes and a black arc for the mouth).

The yawn, Hugo wrote, is the second infectious convulsion of the human face, but the scream must run them a close third (*Man*). In Messerschmidt's "Yawner,"

> the mouth yawns open in a terrible simulation of a scream. We see right into the mouth cavity. We can examine the tongue and its underside, the lappings of flesh beneath it, the teeth. It is all utterly unseemly, if not grotesque. The chin is pushed down deep into the neck, creating thick, rubberized ripplings of flesh. The neck barely exists at all (Glover).

Screams occur during momentous life events like childbirth or orgasm and moments of terror or anguish. They demand an urgent or empathetic response. Allen Ginsberg, writing in 1955, responded to the suffering caused by Moloch-capitalism with a "howl" of rage and pain, a descendant of Walt Whitman's "barbaric yawp." In a 1936 letter to Jean

Paulhan from Mexico, Artaud described how his work as an actor was linked with a primal roar – of "bringing up my fear in the noise of rage, in a solemn roar." Artaud described his screams as an attempt at a "cry as if it came from the bottom of the abyss itself" (Barber). When Arthur Janov tried to get his patients to call for their parents, they would become extremely emotional and eventually produce an uncanny scream, a scream he identified as the voice of a universal neurotic pain. The German psychologist Hilarion Petzold defined the scream as the psychic outlet for the experiences that affected western industrial societies at the time of the appearance of alternative cultures in the 1970s and 80s: "ecological destruction" and nuclear armament (Kutschke 72).

For Catherine Clément, the scream "does violence to the throat, which is suddenly turned into a hole, as if there were no other way out but to break through a wall" (9). In screaming, the mouth is "no longer a particular organ, but the hole through which the entire body escapes, and from which the flesh descends" (Deleuze 2002:19). The scream, Michel Chion has said, is a crack in time (68).

Mladen Dolar and Douglas Kahn regard the scream as a communication, "speech in its minimal function: an address and an enunciation" (Dolar 2006:28). Although screaming does not engage language, Kahn writes, a parent knows when a child's scream becomes an alarm, while people walk by the screams coming from the roller coaster rides at carnivals (Kahn 345). Emil Hrvatin disagrees: the "scream is not an act which would convey something that language cannot; rather it conveys directly that language cannot convey anything (any more)" (86). Artaud frequently conflates the mouth and anus, calling glottal sounds the "anal tongue" (Scheer 157).

The scream is one of the most basic vocal expressions and the infant can use it right after birth. The child's first scream, according to Hrvatin, is a pure vocalization of inner discontent which the mother interprets as a sign of a hunger, a thirst, etc. "The first scream does not belong to a symbolic order, a child is not yet in a language (the Latin *in-fans* means 'who does not speak'). The scream is not directly addressed to a certain person, but it is dispatched, transmitted, delivered--in order to be *heard!*" (Hrvatin 85-6). The mother's response inscribes the scream into the symbolic order. The second scream, however, is a call, a demand for the mother's presence.

Hermann Bahr reserved the scream as the symbol of the expressionist epoch, of which Munch's "The Scream" can stand as exemplar (Głuchowska

187). Although it came to its title belatedly, Munch described its genesis as follows:

> I was walking along the road with two friends. The sun set. I felt a tinge of melancholy. Suddenly the sky became a bloody red. I stopped, leaned against the railing, dead tired and I looked at the flaming clouds that hung like blood and a sword over the blue-black fjord and city. My friends walked on. I stood there, trembling with fright. And I felt a loud, unending scream piercing nature (Hearn) (6).

This powerful sound seems to reshape the physiology of the central figure: "The distorted shape of the skull-like, hairless head, with its almost featureless face" (Heller 90). The background of the painting is the writing of the scream across time and space, "on the one hand filling it and on the other emptying it, nullifying it" (Hrvatin 90) (8).

So many of Bacon's characters are screaming: the "Study after Velázquez's Portrait of Pope Innocent X," a copy of Diego Velázquez' portrait of Pope Innocent X, shows the sombre face of the subject replaced by a screaming mask. "Screaming Woman" (1925) and "Study for the Nurse in the film *Battleship Potemkin*" isolate one of Bacon's obsessive images: the face of the governess in the Eisenstein, mouth wide open, beginning to scream, although no external horror is depicted or suggested. "I did hope one day to make the best painting of the human cry. I was not able to do it and it's much better in the Eisenstein and there it is" (Stiles 199) (7).

Dolar attempts to negotiate the distance (vast but surprisingly intimate) between the scream and music: "Fascination with the highest female voice, best heard in coloraturas, has its origin probably in nearness of the scream. We could look at coloraturas as tamed, familiarized, aesthetically elaborated screams" (Hrvatin 85). Screams occur in almost all of Wagner's mature operas, and he identified them as an "aural manifestation of Schopenhauer's Universal Will and it is from this element that the art of music eventually derives . . . . The scream is the most obvious sign of existential Angst, the principal subject matter of German expressionist painters and writers" (Friedheim 67 and 70).

The scream is almost always female; the scream in opera is "exclusively female" according to Michel Poizat. Michel Chion and Angelica Fenner, on the other hand, distinguish between a male scream (that of Tarzan) and a female scream (a "shout" as opposed to a "scream"): the first between a male "ostentation of power" and exercise of will and the "'black hole' of female pleasure, which is unspeakable, unthinkable." For Fenner "a man's shout is regarded as exercising will and thereby delineating the boundaries of the self, while a woman's scream becomes associated with limitlessness and the dissolution of self" (Hrvatin 86 and Dixon 438).

In Stanislaw Przybyszewski's novel *The Scream,* an artist, Gasztowt, stops a prostitute from committing suicide. Her scream awakens in him a desire to paint a picture depicting an equivalent to that primitive, animalistic sound. Because he does not manage to remember the sound, he murders the woman to hear it again. This anticipates the story of Brian De Palma's *Blow Out*. The film begins in a screening room where the dailies of a horror film ("Co-Ed Frenzy," where all that are required of the auditioning actors are "tits and a scream") are being reviewed. The sound effects technician Jack Terry (John Travolta) finds the recorded screams unsatisfactory; only the real thing will do and by the end of the film he has captured Sally's (Nancy Allen's) authentic scream as the villain strangles her, a scream that delights the film director but rings hauntingly in Jack's ears long after the event.

The screaming woman of American horror films has been dubbed the "Scream Queen" and, by Carol Clover, the "final girl." At the head of a legion of Scream Queens (including Fay Wray and Barbara Steele), stands Jamie Leigh Curtis, whose scream in *Halloween* as she is murdered remains at high volume until the very last slice of the knife. The final girl, again Curtis, is the one who encounters the mutilated bodies of her friends and witnesses the horror to its full extent. She is chased, cornered, wounded; she screams, staggers, falls, rises to scream again.

Notes

Introduction

1. The writings of the 13th century Andalusian mystic, Ibn Arabi, described a human who is "wholly a face" and who could thus "face" God in every position or posture, whichever direction he takes (El Khachab 133).

2. On the other hand, Adrian Daub writes,

> There's a fair amount of evidence that the technology is nowhere near where it would need to be to realize our Orwellian nightmares. China's Face software requires a passerby to stand still for a few seconds to confirm an ID, not the most likely event in the process of pursuing a criminal. Amazon's facial-recognition software recently matched 28 Members of Congress to digitized mugshots very much not of those 28 Members of Congress.

3. "The quality of multiple reflections that the modern city provides us with has turned it into the natural medium of haunting" wrote the Russian occultist M. V. Pogorelsky. Tom Gunning traces this uncanny effect to the reflections made possible by the manufacture of sheet glass in turn-of-the-century shop windows: "Store windows and mirrors greeted passersby on busy streets, endowing them with optical doubles, mixing passing crowds with their visual phantoms" (Fraser 486-7).

4. In *The Face on the Screen*, Therese Davis deals with this spread diachornically, charting the demystification of the face from the high of Béla Balázs's transcendental cinema closeups to the commercial face contagion of the present.

5. Conversely, in a painting like Archimboldo's *Wasser*, what is revealed is a swarm of aquatic creatures until one steps back far enough for it to become a human face.

Facials 1

1. This trope can be traced back to a passage in Edmund Burke's *A Philosophical*

Inquiry into the Origin of Our Ideas of the Beautiful and the Sublime (1756), to a curious story about the celebrated physiognomist Tommaso Campanella:

> This man, it seems, had not only made very accurate observations on human faces, but was very expert in mimicking such as were any way remarkable. When he had a mind to penetrate into the inclinations of those he had to deal with, he composed his face, his gestures, and his whole body, as nearly as he could into the exact similitude of the person he intended to examine; and thus carefully observed what turn of mind he seemed to acquire by this change. So that, says my author, he was able to enter into the dispositions and thoughts of people as effectually as if he had been changed into the very men.

2. The narrator is able to impute dishonesty to a person by virtue of "their voluminousness of wristband, and their air of excessive frankness."

3. Many commentators have insisted that the face Levinas is working with is not the physical object that sits on our necks: it is "the emblem of the appearance of the idea of infinity that exists within the subject that fundamentally resists comprehension" (Simmons 133). As Levinas himself admits, "the face is not in front of me, but above me" (Butler 131). '"The face, then,'" Alex Danchev writes, "'is not the colour of the eyes, the shape of the nose, the ruddiness of the cheek.' The face may be a face--a human face--but it may also be another part of the body, perhaps even a body part. In *Life and Fate*, as Levinas saw it, the face is the back, or the nape of the neck."

> Throughout a long philosophical lifetime, Levinas was often pressed to explain precisely what he meant by the face, in his rather abstruse usage. He would demur, he would discourse, he would divagate; but he provided no definitive answer. Towards the end, however, he furnished an illustration of extraordinary imaginative power, a vignette that made a deep impression on him, and became almost a key to his thought. The illustration came from a monumental novel, *Life and Fate* (1980) . . . by Vasily Grossman (1905–1964) . . . . 'The story is of families, wives, and parents of political detainees traveling to the Lubyanka in Moscow for the latest news. A line is formed at the counter, a line where one can see only the backs of others. A woman awaits her turn: "[She] had never thought that the human back could be so expressive, and could convey states of mind in such a penetrating way. Persons approaching the counter had a particular way of craning their neck and their back, their raised shoulders with shoulder blades tense like springs, which seemed to cry, sob, and scream"' (Danchev 118).

4. Nineteenth-century writers, Poe, George Eliot and Hugo also played with the vast contrast between the facial surface and a byzantine interior:

> Most writers--poets in especial--prefer having it understood that they compose by a species of fine frenzy--an ecstatic intuition–and would positively shudder at letting the public take a peep behind the scenes, at the elaborate and vacillating crudities of thought--the true purposes seized only at the last moment- at the innumerable glimpses of idea that arrived not at the maturity of full view–at the fully-matured fancies discarded in despair as unmanageable--at the painful erasures and interpolations--in a word, at the wheels and pinions--the tackle for scene-shifting--the step-ladders, and demon-traps--the cock's feathers, the red paint and the black patches, which, in ninetynine cases out of a hundred, constitute the properties of the literary histrio;

> But this superadded consciousness, wearying and annoying enough when it urged on me the trivial experience of indifferent people, became an intense pain and grief when it seemed to be opening to me the souls of those who were in a close relation to me—when the rational talk, the graceful attentions, the wittily-turned phrases, and the kindly deeds, which used to make the web of their characters, were seen as if thrust asunder by a microscopic vision, that showed all the intermediate frivolities, all the suppressed egoism, all the struggling chaos of puerilities, meanness, vague capricious memories, and indolent make-shift thoughts, from which human words and deeds emerge like leaflets covering a fermenting heap (*Veil*);

and

> Penetrate, at certain hours, past the livid face of a human being who is engaged in reflection, and look behind, gaze into that soul, gaze into that obscurity. There, beneath that external silence, battles of giants, like those recorded in Homer, are in progress; skirmishes of dragons and hydras and swarms of phantoms, as in Milton; visionary circles, as in Dante. What a solemn thing is this infinity which every man bears within him, and which he measures with despair against the caprices of his brain and the actions of his life! (*Miserables*).

And of course, the inmost me also consists of viscera: medieval authors contrasted the possibly deceptive outward beauty of the skin with the inside "understood as a vile jelly, viscous ooze or a storage area for excrement" (Agamben 2000:92). "Take her skin from her face, and thou shalt see all loathsomeness under it . . . . within she is full of filthy phlegm, stinking, putrid, excremental stuff: snot and snivel in her nostrils, spittle in her mouth, water in her eyes, what filth in her brains" (Burton).

5. The distinction is manifest in accounts of headless men in antiquity and remote

parts of the world, displaying the relocation of the face that Wegenstein predicted: the Blemmyes (Herodotus, Pliny) bore their facial features on their chest; Epiphagi (Sir John Mandeville) carried their eyes on their shoulders; and the Anthropophagi were "men whose heads Do grow beneath their shoulders" (*Othello*). Lewis Carroll said that the blemmyes were the inspiration for Humpty Dumpty. See René Magritte's mapping of a woman's naked torso as a face with nipples for eyes.

6. These colors and proportions are of course true for only certain populations: when Henry Johnson is burned in the fire and carried away on a stretcher in Stephen Crane's "Monster," little boys chant "Nigger, nigger, never die,/ Black face and shiny eye."

7. There were exceptions of course, Fielding himself wondered whether physiognomy had been wrongly dismissed as a means of assessing character: "However cunning the Disguise be which Masquerader wears he very rarely escapes the Discovery of an accurate Observer; for Nature, which unwillingly submits to the Imposture, is ever endeavouring to peep and show herself," Addison was on both sides of the question:

> It is an irreparable Injustice we are guilty of towards one another, when we are prejudiced by the Looks and Features of those whom we do not know. How often do we conceive Hatred against a Person of Worth, or fancy a Man to be proud and ill-natured by his Aspect, whom we think we cannot esteem too much when we are acquainted with his real Character?

And

> Every one is in some Degree a Master of that Art which is generally distinguished by the Name of Physiognomy; and naturally forms to himself the Character or Fortune of a Stranger, from the Features and Lineaments of his Face. We are no sooner presented to any one we never saw before, but we are immediately struck with the Idea of a proud, a reserved, an affable, or a good-natured Man; and upon our first going into a Company of Strangers, our Benevolence or Aversion, Awe or Contempt, rises naturally towards several particular Persons before we have heard them speak a single Word, or so much as know who they are.

8. Ironically, the potential for dissimulation is denied by Wilde, the master of masks and lying: "Sin is a thing that writes itself across a man's face. It cannot be concealed. People talk sometimes of secret vices. There are no such things. If a wretched man has a vice, it shows itself in the lines of his mouth, the droop of his eyelids, the moulding of his hands even" (*Gray*).

9. Ekman claims that facial expressions are universal and can be recognized as markers of one of seven basic emotions—anger, contempt, disgust, fear,

happiness, sadness, and surprise.

10. There had been concern since Descartes over whether expression was an effect of the will. Descartes and his successors insisted that the passions were voluntary, but Darwin concluded that most "movements of expression, and all the more important ones . . . cannot be said to depend upon the will" (Geroulanos and Sobieszek 45). After the latter opinion was established, the uncontrolled face began to be seen as pathological.

Facials 2

1. A common conceit is that of the mask which, once put on, can't be taken off–"Your face will freeze that way"–as in the film *Onibaba* by Kaneto Shindo (1964).

2. A series of writers, however, taking the position of the veiled woman, find the situation reversed: "The veil denies men their usual privilege of discerning whomever they desire. By default, the women are in command. The female scrutinizes the male. Her gaze from behind the anonymity of her face veil or niqab is a kind of surveillance that casts her in the dominant position" (Masood 226). The dynamic of the veil is thus dual: from the woman's position it denies men the pleasure of looking, a kind of castration (Scott 159).

3, The veil had been banned before, by Mustafa Kemal Atatürk when he established the Turkish Republic in 1923. Women wearing headscarves were prohibited from attending universities and working as teachers, lawyers, doctors, and public servants.

Facials 3

1. However, as John Berger points out:

> The mirror was often used as a symbol of the vanity of women. The moralizing, however, was hypocritical. You painted a naked woman because you enjoy looking at her, you put a mirror in her hand and you called the painting Vanity, thus morally condemning the woman whose nakedness you had depicted for your own pleasure (51).

2. Jeffrey Peters disagrees:

> The close-up of the human face is not . . . fundamentally an image of

> interiority or subjectivity in contact with an objective world, nor is it a way into the unconscious, as Balázs and, later, Walter Benjamin suggested it was. Instead, it is, in Deleuze's words, an autonomous "entity," or an expression of pure affect (1987:1054).

3. And from Dickens's *A Tale of Two Cities*,

> Over the prisoner's head there was a mirror, to throw the light down upon him. Crowds of the wicked and the wretched had been reflected in it, and had passed from its surface and this earth's together. Haunted in a most ghastly manner that abominable place would have been, if the glass could ever have rendered back its reflections, as the ocean is one day to give up its dead.

In Jean Rhys's, *Good Morning, Midnight*, a lavatory mirror speaks back: "Would you believe me that, of all the faces I see, I remember each one, that I keep a ghost to throw back at each one--lightly, like an echo--when it looks into me again?" (142). In *An Essay Concerning Human Understanding*, John Locke reverses the trope: "The soul in such a state of thinking, does very little, if at all, excel that of a Looking-glass, which constantly receives variety of images, or ideas, but retains none; they disappear and vanish, and there remain no footsteps of them."
4. This is roughly parallel to another basic function of the mirror: to bring the outside inside, particularly the nineteenth-century "spy" mirror that reflects who or what waits outside an apartment. For Benjamin, "mirrors bring the open expanse, the streets, into the café—this too, belongs to the interweaving of spaces, to the spectacle by which the flaneur is ineluctably drawn." "The mirror image functions, then, less as an uncanny double than as what Freud names it, an 'intruder,' a messenger from the outside disrupting the illusion of homey security" (Gunning 126).

5. As in "The Tain," the mirror reflection is often an enemy or a competitor–in Stellan Rye's *Student from Prague* or Hans Christian Andersen's "The Shadow," where the man and his shadow trade places. "The shadow was the master and the master was the shadow." Because the shadow has attracted the attention of a princess and plans to marry her, the man must allow himself to be called a shadow and must never say that he was at one time a man (*Fairy*).

6. Face to face, according to Peter Laslett and Roy Porter, was also a primary social fact that was rendered inaccessible around 1700 due to population growth (Woods).

7. Another common binary is bourgeois/artist:

> Fichte's notion that the subjective ego was immanently capable of infinite self-replication allowed the German Romantics to create

> characters with two selves - the one quotidian, bourgeois, and limited, the other supernatural, demonically creative, and uninhibited. Particularly in the works of E.T.A. Hoffmann, Achim von Arnim, and Jean Paul, the middle-class ego is constricted by rigid social norms, while his or her Doppelgänger tends to be an artistic figure who transcends these barriers to personal development (Pizer 41).

Erasmus Spikher in Hoffmann's "New Year's Eve's Adventure" "exchanges his mirror image, the signifier of bourgeois propriety, for a life of unbridled passion in Italy, the realm of aesthetic decadence" (Chalupa 16).

8. Here are two more formulations:

Stories of the double "protest against and then reenact that drama of insertion into human culture which is the time when, with the acquisition of identity, our many protean selves, our undifferentiated elements, are 'unified' and stabilized as 'one' character," haunting the unitary subject with a reminder of all that has been excluded and amputated in the process of social formation (Jackson).

Susan Sencindiver advances the familiar feminist subversion of the doubling narrative as a covert act of male mothering, pointing out how clearly the pregnant woman doubles the doppelganger: "She houses a second self within, her body splits into two at childbirth, and she undergoes bodily and psychic metamorphosis" (33).

9. Similar mirror scenes can be found in Max Linder's "Seven Years" and Chaplin's "The Floorwalker." In the Linder, the illusion is broken when he looks at the other and, instead of seeing a face and a front, sees a rear and an ass. In the Chaplin the mirror exchange goes on until Chaplin raises a cane while the double raises a satchel.

10. Lacan defines the *objet à* (the unattainable object of desire) as an object "which cannot be grasped in the mirror" since, like vampires, it has no specular image. The object a, the unattainable object of desire always sought in the other. In classic motion picture the screen refuses to reflect what is standing in front of it, the cameraman and his equipment.

11. Adoring one's mirror image is carried over into narratives about twins, about a subject caught up in the search for a lost double, as in John Banville's *Birchwood* and *Mefisto*. Freudian psychoanalyst Dorothy Burlingham argues in "The Fantasy of Having a Twin" that the same emotional situation that produces the "family romance" in which a child fantasizes about being reunited with lost parents also produces a frequent fantasy in singletons for a reunion with a lost twin.

12. Conrad wants it both ways: "He was not a bit like me, really; yet, as we stood leaning over my bed place, whispering side by side, with our dark heads together

and our backs to the door, anybody bold enough to open it stealthily would have been treated to the uncanny sight of a double captain busy talking in whispers with his other self."

13. Both tales are clouded by an over-insistence on the doubling--asserting it repeatedly, weaving it through every narrative turn: a doubling of moods ("The self-possession of that man had somehow induced a corresponding state in myself"), of clothing ("a sleeping suit of the same gray-stripe pattern as the one I was wearing"), of background ("a Conway boy")–an imaginary class tie worn by a naked sailor is necessary to explain the captain's suicidal loyalty to Leggatt at the expense of the rest of the crew.

Cesare Casarino agrees, finding in the tale "a paroxysmal escalation of redoubling"--

> Virtually on each and every remaining page of this text, however, the narrator not only identifies himself with Leggatt ever more insistently and directly through expressions such as "my other self," "my secret self," "my second self," "the secret sharer of my life," "the double captain," "myself," "my very own self," but he also repeatedly presents the question of the double as the crux of his anxiety-ridden narrations--

and decides that what it adds up to is "the narrator's compelling desire to construct Leggatt as his double." As the ship rounds, narrowly escaping utter destruction, the captain exalts in "the perfect communion of a seaman with his first command" (221 and 220).

"William Wilson" exhibits this same insistent doubling, to and beyond the point of self-mockery:

> Perhaps it was this love he showed for me, added to the fact that we had the same name, and also that we had entered the school on the same day, which made people say that we were brothers . . . . I learned that we were both born on the nineteenth of January, eighteen hundred and nine . . . . I had not then discovered the surprising fact that we were of the same age; but I saw that we were of the same height, and I saw that in form and in face we were also much the same.

Balduin in *The Student of Prague* shoots at his reflection who then disappears. Balduin is delighted but when he looks into his hand mirror he sees he has shot himself. In a related figure, Mallarme's Hérodiade flees the world and plunges into her image reflected by the mirror. In Georges Rodenbach's "L'Ami des miroirs," a man attempts to leap into his mirror, breaking it and ending his life in the process. A similar figure is also found in Poe's "The Fall of the House of Usher," when the house falls into its mirror image in the tarn.

14. According to Richard Ashby, in this play "Shakespeare dramatizes the

psychosomatic fallout that takes place when . . . the subject is suddenly denied a reflecting look," but Ashby tells only half the story, the half that fits his Lacanian model (1262). D. W. Winnicutt theorized this authenticating gaze: "only when a subject feels that he or she has been seen by an other, and only through an interaction of gazes with an other, can he or she sense their own separate existence" (Benziman 59).

15. Good and evil twins, promiscuous and chaste twins–for example, *The Whole Town is Talking* (John Ford, 1935), *A Stolen Life* (Paul Czinner, 1939), *Cobra Woman* (Robert Siodmak, 1944), *The Dark Mirror* (Robert Siodmak, 1946), *The Guilty* (John Reinhardt, 1947), *Dead Ringer* (Paul Henreid, 1964), *Killer in the Mirror* (Frank De Felitta, 1986), *Lies of the Twins* (Tim Hunter, 1991), *Mirror Images I* (Gregory Hippolyte, 1991) and *Twin Sisters* (Tom Berry, 1992).

16. "Snapchat" is the "the fun app to Exchange faces" with, along with "Face Swap" and "Face Stealer."

Earlier face exchanges would include the overpainting of George Washington onto the the face of George III in Washington Irving's "Rip Van Winkle" or the priest's house, "in a film by Razumny," with a portrait of Nicholas II hanging on the wall. When the village is taken by the Red Army, the frightened priest turns the portrait over and on the reverse side is the smiling face of Lenin (Kuleshev 54). In Jody Shields's *The Crimson Portrait*, Catherine substitutes the portrait of her dead husband for the original face of a disfigured veteran as a working guide for the portrait-mask maker. Bereft of his beloved, a plastic surgeon, Philip Ritter (Paul Henreid), in Terence Fisher's *A Stolen Face* gives her face to a disfigured petty criminal whom he then marries. Alfred Hitchcock's *Vertigo* performs the same plot cosmetically.

17. Troy-as-Sean faces Sean-as-Troy in prison, and exclaims "God I miss that face," tries to lick it, and Sean explodes in disgust catching him by the throat. Licking faces is Troy's shtick; Sean's is running his hand over the other's face–two ways of verifying that the face is really there.

18. Cindy Jackson is an American woman who holds the world record for the most plastic surgeries, around thirty operations, in an effort to transform herself into that cultural icon of beauty, the Barbie doll, while Michael Jackson had repeated facial operations in order to approximate whiteness. Cosmetic-plastic surgery has also become the basis of reality TV shows like *Extreme Makeover*, *Nip and Tuck*, and *I Want a Famous Face* (where participants are reshaped in the image of their favorite pop idol).

Facials 4

1. In the Napoleonic wars, victims of facial injuries were generally left on the battlefield or killed by their fellows

2. Milan Kundera describes Bacon's art as an assault on the face; Deleuze understands his project as a portrait painter to be one of "dismantling" the face (Deleuze 2002:20-1). The artist told an interviewer that he loathed his face, and in his art he consistently presents "tortured and visceral portraits" with grotesquely split faces (Kemp 57). Although Biernoff denied any connection between Bacon's faces and twentieth-century wars his mutilation has been linked by others to modern violence (Le Moigne 118). Jonathan Jones identified his faces (particularly the third panel of his 1967 triptych "Three Studies for a Self-Portrait") with photographs found in a pictorial history of the first world war. Of course, it can just as easily go the other way, as Desmond Morris writes:

> Others may see in this screaming face a reflection of the agonies of war-torn Europe, a statement about the horrors of modern existence, or the entrapment and isolation of modern man in his urban cell. I see nothing of the sort. I see a devout masochist enjoying the thrill of encapsulating the secret joys of his most private moments (111).

3. Biernoff passes over portraits of wounded soldiers by Henry Tonks (justifiably so; no one, other than doctors, was supposed to see them). Wyndham Lewis's satirical "Tyros" paintings have also been related to the facially wounded of WWI. Sander Gilman reports a similar reluctance to display wounded faces in America: "During the Gilded Age . . . the wounded of the Civil War were rarely described in terms of their facial wounds . . . . Despite the great interest in the photograph as part of the ongoing memorialization during Reconstruction, the representation of the wounded face did not achieve iconic significance" (161).

4. In Beckmann's "The Way Home" (1919), a man (modeled on the artist) assists a maimed and facially disfigured veteran in finding his way. In one of Grosz's best-known paintings, "Gray Day" (1921), a satirically portrayed, well-dressed official turns his back on a faceless worker carrying a shovel. Ernst Friedrich's *War Against War!* published photographs of veterans with gruesome facial wounds; Susan Sontag refers to them as "heartrending, stomach-turning pictures" that together form "the most unbearable pages in [that] book" (Gehrhardt 180). Other instances could include Mr. Peachum as the beggar king dispatching his army of disabled veterans in Bertolt Brecht's *The Threepenny Opera* and Leonhard Frank's last novella, *The War Cripples*.

See also Robert Minor's illustration of a man of iron lacking a head for *Masses*, July 1916, entitled, "At Last a Perfect Soldier." The "mouthless dead" in

Charles Sorley's "When you see millions of the mouthless dead" (1915) are the military recruits molded into "nameless, faceless, subservient subjects" (Ezekiel Black 1-2).

5. There were also exhibits of deformed faces at the Charité in Berlin and at King's Hospital in London. Deformed faces could of course be displayed in the hospitals themselves.

6. The Russian futurists (Vladimir Mayakovsky, David Burliuk, Aleksei Kruchenykh, and Valery Kamensky) used their own faces as painterly canvases . . . . Igor Larionov, the innovator of this practice appeared at the first meeting of a group called "Aesthetics" "with a 'rayonist landscape' drawn in blue, yellow and green on his face." Larionov and Ilia Zdanevich composed the manifesto "Why We Paint Ourselves" in 1913 in which the artists declared that the unadorned face is "vile" (McQuillen 428).

In America, ironically, a phobic reaction to unsightly war-induced injuries, scars, and deformities resulted in a compulsive search for beauty: "mutilation drove beautification" (Lubin 2016:217).

7. The mannequins of this period in de Chirico's art were certainly prompted by his decision to enlist in May 1915; they have tortured expressions and their faces are heavily scarred (Bohn 163).

After returning from World War I in 1918, severely wounded and grieving over parting with Alma Mahler, Oskar Kokoschka turned to the work of dollmakers Lotte Pritzel and Hermine Moos and ordered one in the likeness of his lover. He painted "Doll-ma" several times, but, unable to bear her "incredible thingness," he threw a party and decapitated her (Frank).

8. Man Ray experimented with mannequins in photography around the same time as De Chirico. Eugène Atget photographed store window mannequins, for example, "Store, Avenue des Gobelins, 1925," where the nearest one is headless while the others have respectable bourgeois heads. As part of his duties in organizing the 1938 Surrealist Exhibition, Marcel Duchamp invited all the exhibitors to dress a shop window mannequin. The tailor dummy is the subject of Carlo Carrà's "La camera incantata" (1917). In David Alfaro Siqueiros' "Portrait of W. Kennedy" (1919), Kennedy is standing next to one.

9. Robert A. Sobieszek would erect a boundary between the disintegration and the disappearance of the face in modern art. In his study of modern portrait photography they are two distinct phases separated as the deadpan of Andy Warhol and the expressive disintegration of Cindy Sherman.

10. If one wanted to see the authentic face of a nation, one would leave the city

and search for it in the countryside: “The peasant’s face,” Erna Lendvai-Dircksen wrote, “represented traditional values” (Brückle).

11. A comparable disjunction (after WWII) is the opposition of classic and progressive cinema (cinema of the 1970s and 1980s) in terms of their predilection for ordinary versus ravaged faces (See Kember).

And, at roughly the same time, the practice of description in fiction is giving signs of playing out. Kamila Pawlikowska reports on faces that evade physiognomic descriptions, like this one from Virginia Woolf's *Jacob's Room*: “It was as if a stone were ground to dust; as if white sparks flew from a livid whetstone . . . . This was in his face” (193). “In writers like Don DeLillo,” Charles Baxter adds, “there is the additional suggestion that the individual face simply has no importance anymore, that it is the basis of an antiquarian humanism based on unsound ideas about individualism.”

12. In 1899 Edith Wharton wrote a short story about a portrait painter who couldn’t do the face. George Lillo in “The Portrait” is a true artist–“Your other painters do the surface--he does the depths; they paint the ripples on the pond, he drags the bottom”--and so his portrait of the notorious Alonzo Vard should have been his finest work: “according to your theory--that the significance of his work depends on the significance of the sitter--his portrait of Vard ought to be a masterpiece; and it’s his biggest failure . . . . the portrait was a failure. It was magnificently composed; the technique was dazzling; but the face had been--well, expurgated.”

13. The curse of disfigurement fails to work in *Moby Dick*:

> With much interest I sat watching him. Savage though he was, and hideously marred about the face—at least to my taste—his countenance yet had a something in it which was by no means disagreeable. You cannot hide the soul. Through all his unearthly tattooings, I thought I saw the traces of a simple honest heart; and in his large, deep eyes, fiery black and bold, there seemed tokens of a spirit that would dare a thousand devils.

In another culture, in Myanmar, “Khotho” was admired by his community as a miracle, not in spite of but precisely because of his facial deformity, which made him different and marked him as ‘the Other’ in a special, positive sense. His ‘stigma’ “was considered a sign of his being one of the gods’ chosen ones” (Grabher 25). “As the face with us is chiefly admired for its beauty, so with savages it is the chief seat of mutilation” (Darwin).

14. David Lubin indicts the portrait mask within a larger perspective: as being of “a piece with the ‘big lie’ of the war itself, one more officially sanctioned attempt

to conceal war's brutality behind a false front" (2008:12).

Facials 5

1. John Cromwell's 1945 film version with a screenplay by DeWitt Bodeen and Herman J. Mankiewicz transposes the time to World War II: the opening scene is set on December 7, 1941, but the calendar of Mrs. Minnett, now the landlady rather than a housemaid, is still set at April 6, 1917.

2. The villain of the film, Torsten Barring, is played by Conrad Veidt and brings into play the current war raging in Europe as well as the maimed veteran of World War I: "Veidt's roles presented a 'newfound vulnerability' that spoke to the conditions soldiers faced on the home front following the First World War, 'his acting enabled mourning for the losses of the war, a response to aggressive militarized masculinity, and reflections on new forms of modern manhood'" (Hausmann 138). Not an institution to pass up an opportunity for double coding, film also represents Vedit as the proto-Nazi. Set in Sweden, the country of neutrality, Veidt accepts the scarred Anna as his tool and when she is unable to kill a child, accuses her of having a love for the weak and unimportant. Veidt had seen "the real Anna–conqueror, empress," and boasts: "What others have done in other countries, I can do here. The world belongs to the devil. I know how to serve him if I can only get the power."

3. In this chapter I am often confusing ugliness with ugliness in art. Two realms are (or have been) obsessed with beauty: art and heteronormativity.

4. The same binary could of course always be turned to racist ends: In 1793, when Christoph Meiners revised his *Outline of the History of Humanity*, he substituted for the labels of Mongolian and Caucasian the physically descriptive "dark-colored and ugly" and "white, or light-skinned and beautiful" (Hochman 1).

5. Ironically the trope works backwards as well, all old art is ugly too: "Beauty is not the platonically pure beginning but rather something that originated in the renunciation of what was once feared which only in the light of this renunciation became the ugly" (Adorno in Athanassoglou-Kallmyer 33).

6. Beauty and ugliness can also be read as ideal and real, and the new ugly art was appropriately granted the label of "realism."

7. Both the uncanny and the ugly fall under the rubric of the fearful, Gigante writes, but "the crucial distinction between them is that while something may be uncanny for one person and yet not so for another, the ugly is universally

offensive" (567).

8. Cupid is not monstrous (merely invisible), but Venus' initial plan was to make Psyche fall in love with something hideous. Her father was to expect no human son-in-law, but rather a dragon-like creature who harasses the world with fire and iron and is feared by even Jupiter and the inhabitants of the underworld and Psyche's sisters are told that she was lying with the vile winged serpent, who would devour her and her child (Wiki).

9. In Thomas Rowlandson's "Six stages of mending a face," Lady Archer goes through this process in reverse as she makes her morning toilet:

> In the first . . . wearing a night-cap, with unsightly pendent breasts . . . her gaping mouth showing toothless jaws. In the next she fits in an eye, in the third she places a wig on her head, in the fourth . . . she fits in a set of false teeth; in the next she applies rouge to her cheeks with a hare's foot. In the last . . . she appears a pretty young woman.

In Ben Jonson's *Silent Woman*, Ott says of his wife, "A most vile face! and yet she spends me forty pound a year in mercury and hogs-bones. All her teeth were made in the Black-Friars, both her eyebrows in the Strand, and her hair in Silver-street. Every part of the town owns a piece of her." A similar transformation occurs in Poe's "The Spectacles," after the young man looks at his beloved, the most "exquisite I ever beheld" through new glasses:

> Was that- was that- was that rouge? And were those- and were those- were those wrinkles, upon the visage of Eugenie Lalande? And oh! Jupiter, and every one of the gods and goddesses, little and big! what- what- what- what had become of her teeth? "You wretch!" said I, catching my breath- "you- you- you villainous old hag!" "Ag?- ole?- me not so ver ole, after all! Me not one single day more dan de eighty-doo." . . . . By the aid of these, of pearl-powder, of rouge, of false hair, false teeth, and false tournure, as well as of the most skilful modistes of Paris.

Facials 6

1. In the Koran, sinners in Hell have black faces, caused by a fire so fierce that the upper lip of the sinner "is rolled up until it reaches the middle of his head, and his lower lip hangs down until it beats upon his navel" (Lange 431).

2. But the aesthetic taste is immediate too, in one sense: "It is not enough to feel, to be touched confusedly; one must untangle the different nuances; nothing can escape the rapidity of the discernment" (Voltaire in Von Hoffman 142).

3. In the 1985 movie *Mask* by Peter Bogdanovich, Diana, a blind teenage girl, falls in love with Rocky, a boy who has severe facial malformation. When she asks him what he looks like, he jokes that he looks like the Greek Adonis, then says, "I don't really look like Adonis; I've got this real strange disease, and it makes my face look real unreal." Diana proceeds to touch his face, and eventually says, "You look pretty good to me."

Successors of Hugo's comprachicos keep reappearing in French literature: in Gautier:

> At a respectful distance behind the strange traveler, there stood by a pile of trunks a small groom, a sort of old man of fifteen, a liveried gnome, who looked like one of the dwarfs whom the Chinese patiently bring up in porcelain jars to prevent their growing. His flat face, on which the nose scarcely showed, seemed to have been compressed in earliest childhood;

and Maupassant:

> "She is an abominable woman," he replied, "a regular demon, a being who voluntarily brings into the world deformed, hideous, frightful children, monstrosities, in fact, and then sells them to showmen who exhibit such things . . . . She maimed the little unborn being, cramping it with that frightful corset, and made a monster of it. Its head was squeezed and elongated to a point, and its large eyes seemed popping out of its head"

("Jettatura" and "A Mother of Monsters").

4. Addison devoted an issue of the *Spectator* to grinning matches.

5. The Joker offers various reasons for the condition of his face: that he cut himself to make his disfigured wife feel better, only to have her leave him; or that it resulted from a fall into a factory's pool of toxic chemicals. Heath Ledger's Joker explains that on the night his father gutted his mother, he screamed as he watched the mother's murder. His father asked "Why so serious, son . . . let's put a smile on that face," slashing the child from ear to ear. Quilp in Dickens's *Old Curiosity Shop* also has a "hideous grin over-spreading his face." After his final victory in *A Connecticut Yankee in King Arthur's Court*, Merlin dissolves into "such a delirium of silly laughter . . . that he reeled about like a drunken man, and presently fetched up against one of our wires. His mouth is spread open yet; apparently he is still laughing. I suppose the face will retain that petrified laugh until the corpse

turns to dust."

6. In *The Twilight of the Gods* (1888) Heinrich Heine writes of a "great scream running through nature." The Greek god Pan would periodically surprise travelers with a scream, causing them to feel panic.

7. The image, which marked the condition of the spirit at the turn of the century, had to wait twenty years for its title. The original title of the painting was *Despair,* and it was only after he met Stanislaw Przybyszewsky, who later became a very good friend, that Munch changed the title to *The Scream* (Hrvatin 87).

8. Eisenstein's, Munch's and Bacon's screams are silent, as is the scream of the horse in "Guernica." "The Silent Scream" was an iconic 1984 video, dramatizing the supposed agony suffered by an aborted fetus.

Works cited

Project Gutenberg: Joseph Addison, *The Spectator*; Hans Christian Andersen, *Fairy Tales & Stories*; Honoré de Balzac, *Z. Marcas;* Mary Elizabeth Braddon, *Lady Audley's Secret*; Charlotte Brontë, *Jane Eyre & Villette*; Emily Brontë, *Wuthering Heights*; Thomas Browne, *Works*, vol. 1; Edmund Burke, *Writings & Speeches*, vol. 1; Robert Burton, *Anatomy of Melancholy*; Giacomo Casanova, *Memoirs*; Geoffrey Chaucer, *Canterbury Tales*; Earl of Chesterfield, *Letters to His Son*; Wilkie Collins, *Woman in White*; Joseph Conrad, "Secret Sharer;" Stephen Crane, *Monster and Other Stories*; Charles Darwin, *Descent of Man*; Charles Dickens, *Bleak House*, "Hunted Down," *Old Curiosity Shop & A Tale of Two Cities*; John Donne, *Poems*; Alexandre Dumas, *Man in the Iron Mask*; Charles W. Eliot, *Prefaces & Prologues to Famous Books*; George Eliot, *Lifted Veil*; James G. Fraser, *Golden Bough*; Theophile Gautier, "Jettatura;" Thomas Hardy, *A Group of Noble Dames & Return of the Native*; Nathaniel Hawthorne, "Custom House," *Mosses from an Old Manse*, *House of the Seven Gables*; *Marble Faun*, "Minister's Black Veil," *Passages from American Notebooks*, vol. 1, and *Twice-told Tales*; William Hogarth, *Analysis of Beauty*; James Hogg, *Private Memoirs and Confessions of a Justified Sinner*; Victor Hugo, *Les Misérables*, *Notre Dame de Paris* and *Man Who Laughs*; Washington Irving, "Rip Van Winkle;" Henry James, "Beldonald Holbein," "Jolly Corner," *London Life & Sense of the Past*; Ben Jonson, *Epicoene; Or, Silent Woman*; Gaston Leroux, *Phantom of the Opera*; John Locke, *Essay Concerning Human Understanding*, vol. 1; Richard Lovelace, *Lucasta*; Guy de Maupassant, *Entire Original Short Stories* and *Selections From Writings*, vol. 1; McCullers, Carson, *Heart Is Lonely Hunter*; Herman Melville, *Moby-Dick*; John Milton, *Paradise Lost*; *Minor Poets of Caroline Period*, vol. 3; Michel de Montaigne; *Essays*; Friedrich Nietzsche, *Beyond Good & Evil*, *Dawn of Day & Thus Spoke Zarathustra*; Plato, *Charmides & Timaeus*; Pliny the Elder, *Natural History*, vol 6; Edgar Allan Poe, "Raven and Philosophy of Composition," & *Works*, vols. 1, 2, 3 and 5; Marcel Proust, *Swann's Way*; Samuel Richardson, *Pamela*; John Ruskin, *Modern Painters*, vol. 1 and *Stones of Venice*; Walter Scott, *Guy Mannering*; William Shakespeare, *Comedy of Errors*, *Hamlet*, *Henry* V, 3 *King Henry VI, King Lear*, *Macbeth*, *Othello* and *Romeo and Juliet*; Mary Shelley, *Frankenstein*; Edmund Spenser, *Tales Chosen from the Faerie Queene*; Robert Louis Stevenson, *Merry Men* and "Strange Case of Dr. Jekyll and Mr. Hyde;" Bram Stoker, *Dracula*; *Tales from the German*; Theocritus, *Translations*; Mark Twain, *Connecticut Yankee in King Arthur's Court* and *Tragedy of Pudd'nhead Wilson*; H. G. Wells, *Invisible Man* and *Island of Dr. Moreau*; Edith Wharton, *Crucial Instances*; Oscar Wilde, *Duchess of*

Padua, Intentions & Picture of Dorian Gray; Émile Zola. *Nana.*

Wikipedia. Cupid and Psyche; *Gueules Cassées*; Kuleshov Effect; Persona and Ugly Law.

Abe, Kōbō. *Face of Another*. Harmondsworth: Penguin, 1972.

Adorno, Theodor. *Quasi una Fantasia: Essays on Modern Music*. NY: Verso, 1992.

Agamben, Giorgio. Infancy and History. NY: Verso, 1993.
Means without End. Mpls: MNUP, 2000.

Alexander, Caroline. "Faces of War." *Smithsonian Magazine*, 2007. Online.

Alvarez, Al. *Savage God.* NY: Norton, 1971.

Ashby, Richard. "Face-off: defacement, ethics & 'neighbour' in *Comedy of Errors*." *Textual Practice* 32(8), 2018, 1255-1275.

Athanassoglou-Kallmyer, Nina. "Ugliness." 31-50. In *On Politics of Ugliness*. Cham, Switzerland: Palgrave Macmillan, 2018.

Aumont, Jacques. *Du visage au cinéma.* Paris: Editions de l'Etoile/Cahiers du cinéma, 1992. Translation by Mary Ann Doane.

Baker, Naomi. "'To make love to Deformity.'" *Renaissance Studies* 22(1), 2008, 86-109.

Bakhtin, Mikhail. *Rabelais & His World.* Bloomingdale: UINDP, 1984.

Baqué, Dominique. "Face as Enigma." *Art-Press* 317, 2005, 42-52.

Barber, Stephen. "Foundry of the Figure." 1987. Online.

Barthes, Roland. *Camera Lucida*. NY: Hill & Wang, 1981.
"Face of Garbo." *Mythologies*. NY: *Ibid.*, 1972.

Basu, Srimati. "V Is for Veil, V Is for Ventriloquism." *Frontiers* 31(1), 2010, 31-62.

Baudelaire, Charles. "In Praise of Cosmetics." Online.

Baudrillard, Jean. *System of Objects*. London: Verso, 1996.

Baxter, Charles. "Loss of Face." 2003. Online.

Beerbohm, Max, "Defense of Cosmetics." Online. 1894.

Belting, Hans. *Face & Mask*. PrincetonUP, 2017.

Benjamin, Walter. *Illuminations*. London: Pimlico, 1999.
Work of Art in Age of Its Technological Reproducibility, & Other Writings on Media. Belknap Press of Harvard UP, 2008.

Benson, Peter & Kevin O'Neill. "Facing Risk." *Anthropology of Consciousness* 18(2), 2007, 29–55.

Benziman, Galia. "Dispersed Are We." *Journal of Narrative Theory* 36(1), 2006, 53-71.

Berger, Anne-Emmanuelle. "Newly Veiled Woman." *diacritics* 28(1), 1998, 93-119.

Berger, Jr., Harry. *Fictions of the Pose*. StanfordUP, 2000.

Berger, John. *Ways of Seeing*. NY: Viking Press, 1972.

Berman, Patricia G. *James Ensor: Christ's Entry into Brussels in 1889*. LA: Getty 2002.

Biernoff, Suzannah. *Portraits of Violence*. Ann Arbor: UMIP, 2017.
"Rhetoric of Disfigurement in First World War Britain." *Social History of Medicine* 24(3), 2011, 666–685.

Biro, Matthew. *Dada Cyborg*.

Black, Daniel. "What Is a Face?" *Body & Society* 17(4), 2011, 1-25.

Black, Ezekiel. "Mouthlessness and Ineffability in World War I Poetry and *The Waste Land*." *War, Literature, & Arts* 25, 2013, 1-17.

Blas, Zach. "Escaping the Face: Biometric Facial Recognition and Facial Weaponization Suite." 2013. Online.

Bonfante, Larissa. "Fraud and the Psychoanalytical Meaning of the Baubo Gestures in Ancient Art." *Notes on the History of Art* 27 (2/3), 2008, 2–9.

Borges, Jorge Luis. "Fauna of Mirrors." 1974. Online.

Bozovic, Miran. "Diderot on Nature and Pantomime." *European Legacy* 23(6), 2018, 643-657.

Boyd, Nolan. "Warped Mirror." *Disability & Society* 31(10), 2016, 1321-1332.

Bray, Joe. "Language of Portraiture in the Early Nineteenth-century Novel." *Women's Writing*, 23(1), 2016, 53-67.

Bray, Patricia L. *Street View*. 2011. Online.

Brilliant, Richard. *Portraiture*. London: Reaktion, 1991.

Brink-Roby, Heather. "Psyche: Mirror & Mind in *Vanity Fair*." *ELH* 80(1), 2013, 125-147.

Brisini, Travis. "Practice of Smiling." *Text and Performance Quarterly* 37(1), 2017, 1-19.

Brophy, John, *Face In Western Art*. London: Harrap, 1963.

Brown, Carol. *James Ensor 1860-1949*. London: Lund Humphries, 1997.

Brückle, Wolfgang. "Face-Off in Weimar Culture." 2013. Online.

Brunel, Pierre. *Companion to Literary Myths, Heroes & Archetypes*. NY: Routledge, 1996.

Bruns, Gerald L. "What's in a Mirror: James Joyce's Phenomenology of Perception." *James Joyce Quarterly* 49(3/4), 2012, 573-588.

Burlingham, Dorothy."Fantasy of Having a Twin." *Psychoanalytic Study of the Child* 1(1), 1945, 205-10.

Butler, Andrew M. "Tain & the Tain." *New Centennial Review* 13(2), 2013, 133-153.

Butler, Judith. *Precarious Life*. NY: Verso, 2004.

Campbell, Joseph. *Mythic Image*. PrincetonUP, 1974.

Cante, Richard C. "Gay Face (and Its Abilities)." *Trans-Scripts* 4, 2014, 111-38.

Carcopino, Jerome. *Daily Life in Ancient Rome*. New Haven, MA: YaleUP, 1940

Carrier, David. “Methodologies & Theory, Old and New.” *Art Journal* 56(2), 1997, 93-5.

Carter, Angela. *Bloody Chamber*. NY: Penguin, 1979.

Casarino, Cesare. “The Sublime of the Closet.” *Boundary 2* 24(2), 1997, 199-243.

Castiglione, Baldassare. *The Book of the Courtier*. Online.

Cather, Willa. “The Portrait.” Online.

Causey, Andrew. “Jacob Epstein’s *Rock Drill*.” 78-100. In *London, Modernism, and 1914*. NY: Cambridge UP, 2010.

Chadwick, Whitney. “Fetishizing Fashion/Fetishizing Culture.” 294-In *Women in Dada*. Cambridge, MA: MITP, 1998.

Challamel, M. Augustin. *The History of Fashion in France*. 1882. Online.

Chalupa, Cynthia. “Re-Imaging the Fantastic.” *Marvels & Tales* 20(1), 2006, 11-29.

Charalampous, Charis. “The Mirror and the Lover’s ‘I’ in Shakespeare’s Sonnets.” *Early Modern Literary Studies* 20(1), 2018, 1-21.

Chatzopoulos, Giorgios. “Os and Bucca.” 2018. Online.

Chaouli, Michel. “Devouring Metaphor.” *The German Quarterly* 69(2), 1996, 125-143.

Chion, Michel. *The Voice in Cinema*. NY: ColumbiaUP, 1982.

Clément, Catherine. *Syncope*. Mpls: UMNP, 1994.

Clover, Carol. “Her Body, Himself.” *Representations* 20, 1987, 187-228.

Coates, Paul. *Screening the Face*. London: Palgrave Macmillan, 2012.

Cole, Jonathan. *About Face*. London: MIT Press, 1999.

Coleman, Simon. “On Mauss, Masks, and Gifts.” 2015. Online.

Conley. Tom. “Faciality.” 101-2. *The Deleuze Dictionary*. EdinburghUP, 2010.

Cousins, Mark. “The Ugly, Part 1.” *AA Files* 28, 1994, 61-64.

"Part 2." 29, 1995, 3-6.

Craft, Christopher. "Come See About Me." *Representations* 91(1), 2005), 109-136.

Crary, Jonathan. *Suspensions of Perception*. Cambridge, MA: MITP, 2001.

Crivelli, Carlo and Allan J. Fridland. "Facial Displays Are Tools for Social Influence." *Trends in Cognitive Sciences* 22(5), 2018, 388-99.

Dalle Vacche, Angela. "Surrealism in Art and Film." 181-97. In *Global Art Cinema*. NY OxfordUP, 2010.

Danchev, Alex. "War Photography, the Face, and Small Acts of Senseless Kindness." *Journal for Cultural Research* 15(2), 2011, 113-29.

Daub, Adrian. "The Return of the Face." 2018. Online.

Davis, Nick. "The Face Is a Politics." *Camera Obscura* 29(2), 2014, 149–183.

Davis, Therese. *The Face on the Screen*. Portland, OR: Intellect, 2004.

Davison, Francis. *Poetical Rhapsody*. London: George Bell & Sons, 1890.

Dean, Carolyn J. Review of Amy Lyford, *Surrealist Masculinities*. *H-France Review* 9 (#45), 2009, 177-80.

Deleuze, Gilles. *Cinema 1: The Movement Image*. NY: Athlone, 1989.
Francis Bacon. Minneapolis: MNUP, 2002.
and Félix Guattari. *A Thousand Plateaus*. MNUP, 1987.

DeNitto, Dennis. "Jean Cocteau's Beauty and the Beast." *American Imago* 33, 1976, 123-54.

Deppman, Hsiu-Chuang. "Rereading the Mirror Image." *Journal of Narrative Theory* 31(1), 2001, 31-64.

Diderot, Denis. *On Art*, New Haven: Yale UP, 1995.

Ding, Katherine. "The Legible Face and the Illegible Body." *ELH* 85(3), 2018, 715-746.

Dixon, Deborah P. "Scream." *Cultural Geographies* 18(4). 2011, 435–455.

Doherty, Brigid. "Figures of the Pseudorevolution." *October* 84, 1998, 64-89.

Dolan, Frances E. "Taking the Pencil out of God's Hand" PMLA 108(2), 1993, 224-239.

Dolar, Mladen. "I Shall Be with You on Your Wedding-Night." *October* 58, 1991, 5-23.
A Voice and Nothing More. Cambridge, MITP, 2006.

Dolezal, Luna. "Cosmetic Surgery as 'Cut-Up.'" 2018. Online.

Dostoevsky, Fyodor. *The Double*. Richmond, Surrey: Alma, 2013.

Drew-Bear, Annette. *Painted Faces on the Renaissance Stage*. Lewisburg, PA: BucknellUP, 1994.

Dufay, Sébastien. "*Retrouver la Face*." 121-132. In *Visage et Portrait, Visage ou Portrait. Presses universitaires de Paris Nanterre*, 2010.

de Fren, Allison. "The Anatomical Gaze in Tomorrow's Eve." *Science Fiction Studies* 36(2), 2009, 235-265.

Eddington, A. S. *The Nature of the Physical World*. Cambridge UP, 1929.

Elias, Norbert. "Essay on Laughter." *Critical Inquiry* 43, 2017, 281-304.

El Khachab, Walid. "Face of the Human and Surface of the World Reflections on Cinematic Pantheism." Online.

Emrali, Refa. "Surrealist Inheritance in Drawing." 2015. Online.

Fanon, Frantz. *A Dying Colonialism*. NY: Grove Press, 1967.

Fara, Patricia. *Sympathetic Attractions*. PrincetonUP, 1996.

Feo, Katherine. "Invisibility: Memory, Masks and Masculinities in the Great War." *Journal of Design History* 20(1), 2007, 17-27.

Fischer, Lucy. "Two-Faced Women." *Cinema Journal* 23(1), 1983, 24-43

Flaig, Paul. "Lacan's Harpo." *Cinema Journal* 50(4), 2011, 98-116.

Flatley, Jonathan. "Warhol Gives Good Face." 101-33. In *Pop Out: Queer Warhol*. Durham, NC: DukeUP, 1993.

Foster, Michael Dylan. "Early Modern Past to Postmodern Future: Changing Discourses of Japanese Monsters." In *The Ashgate Research Companion to Monsters and the Monstrous*. Farnham, Surrey: Ashgate, 2012.

Frank, Priscilla. "The Creepy Tale Of An Artist Who Ordered, Then Decapitated, A Doll Made To Look Like His Ex." 2018. Online.

Fraser, Graham. "The Ghost in the Mirror." *The Modern Language Review* 113(3), 2018, 481-505.

Freud. Sigmund. "The Uncanny." 1919. Online.

Friedberg, Anne. *Window Shopping*. Berkeley: UCAP, 1993.

Friedheim, Philip. "Wagner and the Aesthetics of the Scream." *19th-Century Music* 7(1), 1983, 63–70.

Friend, David. "World War One: Soldiers helped at Wandsworth 'Tin Noses Shop.'" 2014. Online.

Frow, John. *Character and Person*. OxfordUP, 2014.

Garner Jr., Stanton B. "The Gas Heart : Disfigurement and the Dada Body." *Modern Drama* 50(4), 2007, 500-516.

Gascoigne, Laura. "Art for Dummies: an exhibition documenting the role of the mannequin in art history is a revelation." 2014, Online.

Gerhardt, Marjorie. *Men With Broken Faces*. NY: Peter Lang, 2015.

Geroulanos, Stefanos. "Francois Delaporte: Anatomy of the Passions." Online.

Gigante, Denise. "Facing the Ugly." *elh* 67(2), 2000, 565-587.

Gilbert, Sandra and Susan Gubar. *The Madwoman in the Attic*. New Haven: YaleUP, 1979.

Gilman, Sander. *Making the Body Beautiful*. Princeton UP, 1999.

Gitelman, Lisa. "*Emoji Dick* and the Eponymous Whale." 2018. Online.

Glover, Michael. "Great Works: The Yawner." 2011. Online.

Głuchowska, Lidia. Munch, Przybyszewski and The Scream. 2013. Online.

Goffman, Erving. *Interaction Ritual*. NY: Anchor, 1967.

Gogol, Nikolai. "The Portrait." Online.

Goldstein, David B. 75-92. In *Shakespeare and the Power of the Face*. Burlington, VT: Ashgate, 2015.

Gombrich, E. H. *Art, Perception, and Reality*. Baltimore: JHUP, 1972.

Grabher, Gudrun M. *Levinas and the Other in Narratives of Facial Disfigurement*. London: Routledge, 2019.

Graham, John. "Lavater's *Physiognomy*: a Checklist." *Papers of the Bibliographical Society of America* 55(4), 1961, 297-308.

Gregor, Joseph *Masks of the World*. Mineola, NY: Dover, 1936.

Grinnell, George C. "Veiling and Other Fantasies of Visibility." *The New Centennial Review* 13(3), 2013, 241-266.

Gumport, Elizabeth. "INTERIORS: Art and War in Pat Barker's 'Noonday.'" *New Yorker* 2016. Online.

Gunning, Tom. "The Exterior as Intérieur." *Boundary 2* 30(1), 2003, 105-29.

Gural, Natasha. "Unmasking James Ensor." 2009. Online.

Güven, Samet. "The Image of Veil in Leila Ahmed's Women and Gender in Islam." *Journal of History Culture and Art Research* 2(2), 2013, 88-94.

Guyer, Sara. "Buccality." 77-104. In *Derrida, Deleuze, Psychoanalysis*. NY: Columbia UP, 2007.

Guzlowski, John Zbigniew. "The Assault on Character in the Novels of Thomas Pynchon, John Barth, John Hawkes, and William Gaddis." Online.

Hamburger, Jeffrey F. "To Make Women Weep." *RES* 31, 1997, 9-33.

Hausmann, Vincent. "The Hard Shining Brightness of You." *Camera Obscura* 30(2), 2015, 55-87.

Hayon, Kaya Davies. "Faiza Ambah's Mariam and the Embodied Politics of Veiling in France." *Paragraph* 42(3), 2019, 333–350.

Hearn, Michael Patrick. "Edvard Munch: The Modern Life of the Soul." 2006. Online.

Heins, Laura. "The 'Psyche of the White Man' and the Mass Face on Film." *New German Critique* 43(1), 2016, 59-89.

Heller, Reinhold. *Munch.* UChiP, 1984.

Herzog, Amy. "Suspended Gestures." 63-74. In *Deleuze and the Schizoanalysis of Cinema.* NY: Continuum, 2008.

Hess, Thomas B. *De Kooning.* NY: Walker & Co., 1967.

Hesse, Herman. *Steppenwolf.* London: Picador, 2013.

Hochman, Leah. *The Ugliness of Moses Mendelssohn.* NY: Routledge, 2014.

Hoffmann, E. T. A. *Tales.* UChicagoP, 1969.

Homer. *Iliad.* London: Pan Macmillan, 2020.

"How Cézanne helped invent the modern portrait." 2017. Online.

Howell, Michael and Peter Ford. *The True History of the Elephant Man.* NY: Skyhorse Publishing, 2010.

Hrvatin, Emil. "The Scream." *Performance Research* 2(1), 1997, 82-91.

Jackson, Rosemary. "Narcissism and Beyond." Online.

Jaeger, C. Stephen. "The Redemptive Power of the Face." *Postmedieval* s 8, 2017, 67–82.

James, Henry. *The Portable Henry James.* NY: Penguin Books, 2004.

Jay, Martin. *Downcast Eyes.* Berkeley, UCAP, 1993.

Jones, Colin. *The Smile Revolution in Eighteenth-Century Paris.* OxfordUP, 2014.

Jones, Jonathan. "The beast within." *Guardian*, Aug. 9, 2005, online.

Kahn, Douglas. *Noise, Water, Meat.* Cambridge, MA: MITP, 1999.

Kaiser, Matthew. "Pater's Mouth." *Victorian Literature and Culture* 39(1), 2011, 47-64.

Karim-Cooper, Farah. "Fashioning the Face." 29-42. In *Shakespeare and the Power of the Face*. NY: Routledge, 2015.

Kember, Joe. "David Lynch and the Mug Shot." 29-34. In *The Cinema of David Lynch*. London: Wallflower, 2004.

Kemp, Sandra. "'Myra, Myra on the wall': The fascination of faces." *Critical Quarterly* 40(1), 2004, 38-69.

Kerr, Matthew L. Newsom. "An Alteration in the Human Countenance." 129-46. In *A Medical History of Skin*. Routledge, 2013.

Kessler, Marni Reva. *Sheer Presence*. Mpls.: UMNP, 2006.

Kittler, Friedrich. *Literature, Media, Information Systems*. Amsterdam: OPA, 1997.

Klein, John. *Matisse Portraits*. New Haven: YaleUP, 2001.

Krečič, Jela and Slavoj Žižek. "Ugly, Creepy, Disgusting, and Other Modes of Abjection." *Critical Inquiry* 43(1), 2016, 60-83.

Krips, Henry. "The Hijab, the Veil, and Sexuation." *Psychoanalysis, Culture & Society* 13(1), 35-47. 2008.

Kuleshov, Lev. *Kuleshov on Film*. Berkeley: UCAP, 1974.

Kundera, Milan. "The Painter's Brutal Gesture." 8-18. In *Bacon: Portraits and Self-portraits*. London: Thames and Hudson, 1996.

Kutschke, Beate. "The Scream in Avant-Garde Music." 61-80. In *The Modernist Legacy*. London: Ashgate, 2005.

Lange, Christian. "On That Day When Faces Will Be White or Black." *Journal of the American Oriental Society* 127(4), 2007, 429-445.

Lavater, Johann Caspar. *Essays on Physiognomy*. London: William Tegg, 1878.

Lee, Hermione. "Toby's Room by Pat Barker." 2012. Online.

Le Moigne, Cyrille. "The wrecking of the face." *Beaux Arts Magazine* 292, Oct., 2008, 118-119.

Lennard, Debra. "Censored Flesh." *The British Art Journal* 12(2), 2011, 22-33.

Lessing, Gotthold Ephraim. *Laocoon*. Internet Archive, online.

Levinas, Emmanuel. *Difficult Freedom*. Baltimore, MD: JHUP, 1990.
Totality and Infinity. Dordrecht: Kluwer, 1991.

Lopate, Philip, ed. *The Prince of Minor Writers*. New York Review of Books, 2015.

Lovecraft, H. P. "The Trap." Online.

Lubin, David M. "Masks, Mutilation, and Modernity: Anna Coleman Ladd and the First World War." *Archives of American Art Journal* 47(3/4), 2008, 4-15.

Lyon, John B. "The Science of Sciences." *Eighteenth-century Studies* 40(2), 2007, 257-77.

Maglaque. Erin. "Down With Occurences." *LRB* 3, Dec., 2020, 29-30.

Magli, Patrizia. "The Face and the Soul." 87-127. In *Fragments for a History of the Human Body, Part 2*. NY: Zone, 1989.

Mâle, Emile. *The Gothic Image*. NY: Harper, 1958.

Maley, Barry. "The Burka's Veiled Insult." 2015. Online.

Mansbridge, Joanna. "Fantasies of Exposure." *The Journal of Popular Culture* 49(1), 2016, 29-56.

Marcoci, Roxana. "Perceptions at Play." *Art Journal* 64(4), 2005, 6-25.

Marcus, Laura. *Close Up, 1927-1933*. PrincetonUP, 1998.

Masood, Maliha. "On the Road." 213-227. In *The Veil*. Berkeley: UCAP, 2008.

McLuhan, Marshall. "The Brothel Without Walls." Online.

McQuillen, Colleen. "From 'The Fairground Booth' to Futurism. *The Russian Review*" 71(3), 2012, 413-435.

Meis, Morgan. "Face Off." 2004. Online.

Miéville, China. *Looking for Jake*. NY: Ballantine, 2005.

Miller, J. Hillis. "The Profession of English: An Exchange." *Association of Departments of English Bulletin* 88, 1987, 42-58.

Mishima, Yukio. *Confessions of a Mask*. NY: New Directions, 1958.

Moore, Michael Edward. "Meditations on the Face in the Middle Ages." *Literature and Theology* 24(1), 2010, 19-37.

Morgan, Luke. *The Monster in the Garden*. Phila: UPAP, 2016.

Morris, Desmond, "On Francis Bacon's Three Studies for Figures at the Base of a Crucifixion (c. 1944)." *Tate Etc* 8, 2006, 111.

Murray, Ann. "Reformed Masculinity." 2012. Online.

Nietzsche, Friedrich. *Untimely Meditations*. CambridgeUP, 1983.

Nishimura, Satoshi. "Hardy on Prosopopoeia." *English* 66(252), 2017, 27–39.

O'Bryan, Jill. *Carnal Art*. UMNP, 2005.

Pantazzi, Michael. "A Face of One's Own." *Journal of the Short Story in English* 58, 2012, 201-214,

Pawlikowska, Kamila. *Anti-Portraits: Poetics of the Face in Modern English, Polish and Russian*. Leiden: Brill Rodopi, 2015.

Perpich, Diane. *The Ethics of Emmanuel Levinas*. StanfordUP, 2008.

Peters, Jeffrey N. "Tautou's Face." *PMLA* 126(4), 2011, 1042-1060.

Pinero, Arthur. *The Enchanted Cottage*. London: William Heinemann, 1922.

Pizer, John. "The Kraus/Werfel Polemic: The Double as a Sign of Modernism's Originality Crisis." *Colloquia Germanica* 34(1), 2001, 41-56.

Poore, Carol. *Disability in Twentieth-Century German Culture*. Ann Arbor: UMIP, 2009.

Pop, Andrea and Mechtild Widrich. "Rethinking Ugliness." 2014. Online. *Ugliness*. London: Bloomsbury, 2013.

Porter, Roy. "Making Faces: Physiognomy and Fashion in Eighteenth-Century England." *Etudes Anglaises* 38(4), 1985, 385-396.

Proust, Marcel. *Remembrance of Things Past*: NY: Random House, 1981.

Pultar, Gönül. "Postmodern Resistance or Public Mask." 114-27. In *Post-National Enquiries*. Newcastle Upon Tyne: Cambridge Scholars, 2009.

Pynchon, Thomas. *Gravity's Rainbow*. NY: Viking, 1973.

Rank, Otto. *Beyond Psychology*. NY: Dover, 1941.

Read, Peter. "Picasso and Apollinaire: The Persistence of Memory." Berkeley, UCAP, 2008.

Rhie, Bernie. "Wittgenstein on the Face of a Work of Art." Online.

Rhys, Jean. *Good Morning, Midnight*. London: Penguin, 2000.

Richman, Michèle H. "Spitting Images in Montaigne and Bataille for a Heterological Counterhistory of Sovereignty." *Diacritics* 35(3), 2005, 46-61.

Richter, Gerhard. *Walter Benjamin and the Corpus of Autobiography*. Detroit: Wayne StateUP, 2000.

Rilke, Rainer Maria. *The Notebooks of Malte Laurids Brigge*. NY: Norton, 1949.

Rodrigues, Sara and Ela Przybylo . *On the Politics of Ugliness*. London: Palgrave Macmillan, 2018.

Rodriguez, Mario. "Physiognomy and Freakery." 2014. Online.

Ron, Moshe, "The Art of the Portrait According to James." *Yale French Studies* 69, 1985, 222-237.

Rose, Jacqueline. "Introduction." *Feminine Sexuality*. NY: Norton, 1982.

Rushdie, Salman. *Shame*. London: Cape, 1983.

Rushton, Richard. "What Can a Face Do?" *Cultural Critique* 51, 2002, 219-237.

Saliot, Anne-Gaëlle. *The Drowned Muse*. OxfordUP, 2015.

Sandals, Leah. "A Flight from Face to Face, in Toronto." 2014. Online.

Saramago, José, *The Double*. Orlando: Harcourt, 2004.

Sartre, Jean-Paul. *Nausea*. NY: New Directions, 1964.

Scheer, Edward. *Antonin Artaud: A Critical Reader*. NY: Routledge, 2004.

Schopenhauer, Arthur. *Essays and Aphorisms*. London: Penguin, 1970.

Schor, Naomi. "Blindness as Metaphor." *differences* 11(2), 1999, 76-105.

Schwartz, Hillel. *Culture of the Copy*. NY: Zone, 1996.

Schwyzer, Philip. "Fallen idols, broken noses." *Memory Studies* 11(1), 2018. 21-35.

Scott, Joan Wallach. *The Politics of the Veil*. PrincetonUP, 2007.

Sedgwick, Eve Kosofsky. "The Character in the Veil." *PMLA* 96(2) 1981, 255-270.

Seelig, Beth J. "The Rape of Medusa in the Temple of Athena." The International Journal of Psychoanalysis 83(4), 2002, 895-911.

Sekula, Allan. "The Body and the Archive." *October* 39, 1986. 3–64.

Sencindiver, Susan Yi. "Shared Secrets." *Kontur* 21, 2011, 32-48.

Sennett, Richard. *The Fall of Public Man*. NY: Vintage, 1974.

Serpell, C. Namwali. "[Happy Face]; or, The Word of the Year." 2019. Online.

Shaw, William C. "Social Aspects of Dentofacial Anomalies." 191-216. In *Social and Applied Aspects of Perceiving Faces*. Hillsdale, NJ: Lawrence Erlbaum Associates, 1988.

Siegel, James T. "Georg Simmel Reappears: The Aesthetic Significance of the Face." *Diacritics*, 29(2), 1999, 100-113.

Simmons, Laurence. "Jacques Derrida's Ghostface." *Angelaki* 16:1, 2011, 129-141.

"Sir Gawain and the Loathly Lady." 1985. Online.

"Six stages of mending a face." Online.

Smith, Charles Saumarez. "I Try to Make Everybody Look Great." *Modern Painters* 14(2), 2001, 54-7.

Smith, P. D. "On Reflection." 2004. Online.

Sobieszek, Robert A. *Ghost in the Shell.* LA County Museum of Art, 1999.

Stiles, Kristine. *Theories and Documents of Contemporary Art.* Berkeley: UCAP, 1996.

Stoljar, Margaret. "Mirror and Self in Symbolist and Post-Symbolist Poetry." *The Modern Language Review* 85(2), 1990, 362-372

Strasser, S. "The Smile that Pays." In *The Myth Making Frame of Mind.* Beltom, CA: Wadsworth Publisher, 1993.

Sumera, Laura. "The Mask of Beauty." *Quarterly Review of Film and Video* 26, 2009, 40–46.

Sylvester, David. Interview with De Kooning. In *Willem de Kooning: A centennial exhibition.* NY: Gagosian Gallery, 2004.

Synnott, Anthony. *The Body Social.* London: Routledge, 1993.
"Truth and Goodness, Mirrors and Masks--Part I." *The British Journal of Sociology*, 40(4), 1989, 607- 636.

Tamboukou, Maria. *Nomadic Narratives, Visual Forces.* NY: Peter Lang, 2010.

Taussig, Michael. "Crossing the Face." 224-44. In *Border Fetishisms.* NY: Routledge, 1998.

Teachout. Terry. "What Clement Greenberg Knew." *Commentary*, 2006. Online.

Testimonies to the genius and memory of Sir Joshua Reynolds. 1792. Online.

Thompson Hannah. *Taboo: Corporeal Secrets in Nineteenth-century France.* NY: Modern Humanities Research Association, 2013.

Thorpe, Douglas, "Calvin, Darwin, and the Double." Newsletter of the Victorian Studies Association of Western Canada 11(1), 1985, 6-22.

Tomkins, Silvan. *Affect Imagery Consciousness.* Vol. 1. NY: Springer, 2008.

Toossi, Katayoun Zarei. "The Conundrum of the Veil and Mohja Kahf's Literary Representations of Hijab." *Interventions* 17(5), 2015, 640-656.

Townsend, Christopher. "The Purist Focus." Online.

Tudor, Faye. “All in him selfe as in a glass he sees.” 171-186. In *Renaissance Theories of Vision*. NY: Ashgate, 2010.

Vercelloni, Luca. *The Invention of Taste*. NY: Routledge, 2020.

Vivian, Bradford, “The Veil and the Visible.” *Western Journal of Communication* 63:2, 1999,115-139.

von Hoffmann, Viktoria. “Learning (to) Taste.” *The Senses and Society* 14(2), 2019, 131-147.

Vonnegut, Kurt. *Breakfast of Champions*. NY: Dial, 2011.

Wegenstein, Bernadette. *The Cosmetic Gaze*. Cambridge, MA: MITP, 2012. “Getting Under the Skin, or, How Faces Have Become Obsolete.” *Configurations* 10(2), 2002, 221-259.

Weinberg, Erin. “Not mad, but mated.” *Pacific Coast Philology* 50(2), 2015, 209-225.

Welchman, John C. (Review of *Ghost in the Shell*). The Art Bulletin 83(1), 2001, 161-165.

Welchman, John. “Face[t]s: Notes on Faciality.” *Artforum* 1988. Online.

Werth, Margaret. “Modernity and the Face.” 2006. Online.

West, Nathanael. *Miss Lonelyhearts & The Day of the Locust*. NY: New Directions, 1933.

West, Shearer. *Portraiture*. OxfordUP, 2004.

Wharton, Edith. “The Portrait.” Online.

Whiteley, Giles. *Oscar Wilde and the Simulacrum*. Oxford: Legenda, 2015.

Willette, Jeanne. “Dada in Berlin.” 2019. Online.

Woodall, Joanne, ed. *Portraiture: Facing the Subject*. ManchesterUP, 1997.

Woods, Kathryn. “‘Facing’ Identity in a ‘Faceless’ Society.” *Cultural and Social History* 14(2), 2017, 137-153.

Yeager, Lynn. “The Artists Keeping Up the Tradition of Mask-Making.” 2020. Online.

Ziegler, Robert. *Asymptote: An Approach to Decadent Fiction*. NY: Rodopi, 2009.

Ziolkowski, Jan. "Avatars of Ugliness in Medieval Literature." The Modern Language Review 79(1), 1984, 1-20.

Ziolkowski, Theodore. *Disenchanted Images*. PrincetonUP, 1977.

Žižek, Slavoj, *The Abyss of Freedom*. Ann Arbor: UMIP, 1997.
Disparities. NY: Bloomsbury, 2016.

Zunshine, Lisa. *Introduction to Cognitive Cultural Studies*. Baltimore: JHUP, 2010.

www.ingramcontent.com/pod-product-compliance
Lightning Source LLC
LaVergne TN
LVHW010719210926
848485LV00008B/1453/J
* 9 7 8 1 6 8 0 5 3 7 5 0 5 *